condit

MULTIPLICATION AND DIVISION IN MAMMALIAN CELLS

THE BIOCHEMISTRY OF DISEASE

A Molecular Approach to Cell Pathology

A Series of Monographs

SERIES EDITORS

Emmanuel Farber

Temple University
Philadelphia, Pennsylvania

Henry C. Pitot

McArdle Laboratory for Cancer Research
University of Wisconsin
Madison, Wisconsin

VOLUME 1

The Cell Cycle and Cancer

Edited by Renato Baserga

VOLUME 2

The Pathology of Transcription and Translation

Edited by Emmanuel Farber

VOLUME 3

Molecular Pathology of Connective Tissues

Edited by Ruy Pérez-Tamayo and M. Rojkind

VOLUME 4

Chemical Carcinogenesis (in two parts)

Edited by Paul O. P. Ts'o

and Joseph A. DiPaolo

VOLUME 5

The Liver: Normal and Abnormal Functions

(in two parts)

Edited by Frederick F. Becker

VOLUME 6

Multiplication and Division in Mammalian Cells

Renato Baserga

MULTIPLICATION AND DIVISION IN MAMMALIAN CELLS

Renato Baserga

*Temple University Health
Sciences Center
Philadelphia, Pennsylvania*

MARCEL DEKKER, INC.   New York and Basel

MARCEL DEKKER, INC.
270 Madison Avenue, New York, New York 10016

LIBRARY OF CONGRESS CATALOG CARD NUMBER: 75-25166
ISBN: 0-8247-6353-X

Current Printing (last digit):
10 9 8 7 6 5 4 3 2 1

PRINTED IN THE UNITED STATES OF AMERICA

TO MY DAUGHTERS
SUSAN and JANICE

INTRODUCTION TO THE SERIES

Rudolf Virchow wrote in 1855 as follows:

"When we require cellular pathology to be the basis of the medical view-point, a most concrete and quite empirical task is at stake, in which no a priori or arbitrary speculation is involved. All diseases are in the last analysis reducible to disturbances, either active or passive, or large or small groups of living units, whose functional capacity is altered in accordance with the state of their molecular composition and is thus dependent on physical and chemi-cal changes of their contents. Physical and chemical investigation has a very great significance in this respect, and we can do no more than wish a prosperous development to the school which is striving to form itself. But we should not conceal from ourselves that the story of metabolic interchange will be brought to satisfactory conclusion only when it is carried back to the primary active parts; in other words, when it becomes possible to describe the particular role every tissue, and every pathologically altered part of a tissue, plays in that story. Therefore, although one may begin with the outworks, the ultimate goal, beyond the urine and the sweat and the various waste products of organic activity, must never be lost from sight, nor should it be supposed that these waste products are themselves the goal. There would always be the danger of suffering shipwreck in a more or less exclusively humoral pathology, if this were to be the case."

It has taken a hundred years to start the molecular approach in a fruitful way. Modern developments in physics, chemistry, and mathematics, both conceptual and instrumental, make it now possible to exploit that new-old approach to pathology. Hence, my return to Virchow's expression, cellular pathology.

We, in modern pathology and medicine, are so involved in generating and interpreting the new research available that no one person at this stage could endeavor to write an all-encompassing treatise on the biochemistry of disease. Besides, we do not know enough yet. We can only highlight some of the most interesting details. This will be one of our objectives in this monograph series.

Underlying this are two basic roles of pathology in medicine and biology. The first and most classical role is to analyze disease processes in depth, the aim being as detailed a knowledge as possible about the causes and the cellular and tissue development of disease. Included in this is the production of experimental disease which mimics or simulates the naturally occurring process in order to study it more easily. However, there is a second role which will assume increasing importance as we probe more deeply into cells. The molecular approach to disease has not only as its aim the study of cellular pathology but also the deeper understanding of the normal cell, both structurally and functionally. Through the induction of selected derangements in the cell, especially reversible ones, cellular pathology offers novel but essential ways to dissect the cell. The contributions of the pathologic (genetic, toxic, etc.) in the development of the molecular biology of microorganisms clearly point to an important role for such experimental pathologic systems in the molecular analysis of eukaryotic cells.

All the modern conceptual and methodologic approaches of cellular biochemistry and ultrastructural analysis must be used in such a dissection of the cell. However, our orientation is quite different. Whereas cytochemists nowadays have as their major aim the delineation of the different chemical interactions in cells, the modern cellular pathologist must continually attempt to *integrate* these into a *gestalt* that is meaningful biologically as well as biochemically. Therefore, a second important objective of this monograph series will be the presentation of model systems of higher organisms which are of particular use for the modern biologist interested in the molecular analysis of cell function in higher organisms.

Emmanuel Farber
Philadelphia, Pennsylvania

PREFACE

"If the biologically active substance isolated in highly purified form as the sodium salt of deoxyribonucleic acid actually proves to be the transforming principle, as the available evidence strongly suggests, then nucleic acids of this type must be regarded not merely as structurally important but as functionally active in determining the biochemical activities and specific characteristics of pneumococcal cells." Modern biology began unobtrusively with this statement which appeared in 1944, as the conclusion of a paper by Avery, MacLeod, and McCarty* on the nature of pneumococcal-transforming principle. After Avery, biology has never been the same and it is not surprising that the far-reaching consequences of this statement have also changed our knowledge of cell division, which for a long time has been a favorite but unrewarding topic for the cell biologist. It is this change in our knowledge that I wish to discuss in this monograph, were I will attempt to summarize and arrange in a coherent manner what we know, at this point in time, about cell division in mammalian cells.

Originally trained in the classic precepts of medicine, I have observed with mixed feelings of amusement and nostalgia these classic precepts being replaced, in the last 25 years, by new concepts. Trained in pathology, which was then the official language of medicine, I saw classic morphology slowly lose its position of preeminence, while biochemistry triumphantly emerged as

* Avery, O. T., MacLeod, C. M., and McCarty, M. (1944) J. Exp. Med. 79, 137-158

the new scientific basis of medicine. I, too, went quietly from morphology to biochemistry, something which made me known as an intruder among biochemists, and as a traitor among pathologists. But it is, in fact, this dual background that encourages me to write this monograph in order to show how our knowledge of cell division has gone from the morphological description of mitosis to the molecular basis of the cell cycle. The protagonist of the booklet is the dividing mammalian cell and I will refer to bacteria and lower animals only when necessary for a better understanding of molecular processes.

The monograph is not intended to be an exhaustive source of references, i.e. it is a monograph and not a handbook. I have tried to give preference to those original papers or reviews that have introduced or established certain general concepts. The serious investigator who wishes to know technical details must consult the original works.

I do not apolozige for using extensively my own data, and any reader who wishes to criticize me for that is referred to John 8:7.† At any rate, this monograph is the fruit of long labor and of endless discussions on the literature with associates and friends who have freely given of their time for criticism and suggestions. These colleagues, too numerous to be individually named, I would like to thank at this point. However, I must single out for recognition the students and fellows who have worked with me since 1958, first at Northwestern University and later at Temple University: Richard D. Estensen, Robert O. Petersen, John P. Layde, H. R. Hinrichs, Larry Weiss, Daniel Malamud, Frederick Wiebel, James P. Whitlock, Takehito Sasaki, Luigi Pegoraro, Giovanni Rovera, Gary Stein, Anna Novi, John Farber, Jo Anne Simson, Norbel Galanti, John P. Durham, Atsushi Tsuboi, Leonard H. Augenlicht, Mark Costlow, Sukhen Chaudhuri, Luciano Zardi, Jung-Chung Lin, Bridget T. Hill, Bernd M. Bombik, Claudio Nicolini, Terry Newirth, C. H. Huang, Sandra Whelly, Nancy Chiu, Agnes Kane, Mara Rossini, and Toshinore Ide. Their visible contribution to this monograph is their published work, but of greater importance is their invisible contribution in ideas, criticisms, encouragement, and hard work. To borrow a phrase from an Anonymous longobard chronicler: "In teaching them, my knowledge grew."‡

Renato Baserga

† John, St. (about 120 A.D.) The Gospel, 8:7.

‡ Anonymous (no date) Il Taccuino del Cane Rampante, unpublished manuscript in the Biblioteca della Fata Turchina

CONTENTS

Introduction to the Series   *Emmanuel Farber*   v
Preface   vii

One

**DIVIDING CELLS, NONDIVIDING CELLS,
AND CELLS IN-BETWEEN**   1

    The Cell Cycle   2
    Classification of Cells   5
    The Three Parameters of the Population Explosion   9
    Tumor Growth   11
    References   15

Two

S PHASE   17

    Definition of S Phase   17
    Synchronization of Cells   17
    DNA Synthesis: Factors Required   19
    Asynchronous Replication of Chromosomes   23
    Concomitant Events to DNA Replication   24
    References   28

Three

G$_2$ AND MITOSIS 32

Macromolecular Synthesis in G$_2$ 32
Inhibitors of G$_2$ 33
Length of G$_2$ and Mitosis 34
Membrane Changes in Mitosis 34
Protein Synthesis During Mitosis 37
RNA Synthesis During Mitosis 38
DNA Synthesis and Mitosis 39
References 41

Four

G$_1$ PHASE 44

RNA Synthesis 44
Protein Synthesis 45
Other Biochemical Events 46
Conclusions 49
References 51

Five

THE PREREPLICATIVE PHASE OF G$_0$ CELLS 53

G$_0$ Cells and Bacterial Spores 53
From Mitosis Backward 55
DNA Synthesis 60
The Late Prereplicative Phase 61
The Early Prereplicative Phase 65
From Cyclic Nucleotides to Polyamines 66
A General View of the Prereplicative Phase 69
References 73

Six

GENE ACTIVATION 78

Growth Mutants 78
Definition of the Problem 80
RNA Synthesis and Acitinomycin D 81
Chromatin Template Activity 84
Chromatin Template Activity in Stimulated G$_0$ Cells 88

Changes in Chromatin Structure 92
Appearance of New RNA Species 98
Mechanisms of Increased Transcription 99
References 102

Seven

CHROMOSOMAL PROTEINS 107

Role of Histones in Gene Expression 108
Nonhistone Chromosomal Proteins 113
Nonhistone Chromosomal Proteins and Gene Expression 115
Nonhistone Chromosomal Proteins and Cell Proliferation 117
Chromatin Reconstitution 120
Salt Extraction of Chromatin 124
References 125

Eight

POST-TRANSCRIPTIONAL CONTROLS 131

Types of Post-Transcriptional Controls 131
Modification of Chromatin-associated Proteins 132
Migration to the Nucleus of Preexisting Cytoplasmic
    Proteins 135
De Novo Synthesis of Nonhistone Proteins 138
Inactive mRNA Templates 139
Loss of Cytoplasmic Proteins 142
References 144

Nine

THE ROLE OF MEMBRANES 146

Contact-inhibition of Growth 146
Membrane Changes in Neoplastic Cells 147
Membrane Changes During the Cell Cycle 151
References 156

Ten

GROWTH FACTORS 160

Definition of Growth Factors 160
Stimulatory Factors in Cell Cultures 162

Stimulatory Factors in Animals 167
Inhibitory Factors 168
Mechanism of Inhibition 170
References 172

Eleven

G_0 VERSUS G_1 CELLS 175

Biological Differences 175
Cell Kinetics 178
Differences in Constituent Proteins 180
Transformed and Untransformed Cells 181
Chromatin Template Activity 183
Mechanism of G_0 Transition 184
References 187

Twelve

HYPERTROPHY AND HYPERPLASIA 189

Cell Number and Size 189
Experimental Hypertrophy 191
Molecular Basis of Hypertrophy 194
Growth Induced by Sex Hormones 195
Immunosuppressive Agents 196
RNA 197
References 197

Thirteen

THE CANCER CELL 200

Tumor Growth at the Cellular Level 201
Progression of Tumors 205
The Case of Xeroderma Pigmentosum 206
Viral Transformation 209
References 213

Author Index 215

Subject Index 233

MULTIPLICATION AND DIVISION IN MAMMALIAN CELLS

ONE

DIVIDING CELLS, NONDIVIDING CELLS, AND CELLS IN-BETWEEN

Like La Belle au Bois Dormant, the study of cell division slept for a hundred years after mitosis was first discovered back in 1826. It was Rusconi (1826) who first described segmentation in the ova of frogs and salamanders, thus laying the foundations for the study of cell proliferation, but it was only with the complete description of karyokinesis by Mayzel (1875) that mitosis became firmly established in medicine and biology. This was followed by countless descriptions of the cytological aspects of mitosis in its classic four stages by now familiar to every high school student: prophase, metaphase, anaphase, and telophase. Some perceptive observers, noticing that during mitosis the nuclear material was equally divided between the two daughter cells, even suggested that the genetic material of the cell might be encoded in the nucleus and more specifically in the chromosomes. However, throughout this long period very little was known of the biochemical basis of mitosis and even less of the biochemical events occurring during interphase, that is, during the long interval between two successive mitoses. The situation was summarized as recently as 1950 in a book by Cowdry who, in a discussion of cell division, could devote several pages to a cytological description of mitosis and just a few lines to interphase. Because biochemical information was not available, Cowdry (1950) divided cell populations in the adult animal on a histological basis and in terms of their ability to proliferate into three categories, namely: (a) vegetative inter-mitotics, in which mitoses were frequently found under physiological conditions, as in the lining epithelium of the crypts of the small intestine, some cells of the bone marrow, and the basal layer of the epidermis; (b) reverting postmitotics, for instance, liver and kidney cells, in which mitoses were exceedingly rare but could markedly increase in number if the tissue was stimulated to grow; and (c) fixed postmitotic, like neurons, polymorphonuclear leuko-cytes, keratinizing cells of the epidermis, and so forth, in which mitoses were never found. A consideration of biochemical charac-teristics was thus absent from Cowdry's classification of cell popu-lations, which was based instead on the presence of mitoses as the only available criterion for distinguishing proliferating cells from nonproliferating cells.

THE CELL CYCLE

The first breakthrough in the biochemical wall occurred in 1951 when Howard and Pelc described the rough outlines of the cell cycle in roots of *Vicia faba* seedlings. Using [^{32}P] as a label, Howard and Pelc were able to show that DNA was synthesized in a discrete period of the interphase preceding mitosis, the first demonstration of a specific biochemical event occurring in inter-phase and related to cell division. By that time, the work of Avery et al. (1944) and Hershey and Chase (1952) had pointed to DNA as the most likely candidate for genetic material, and the findings of Howard and Pelc (1951) therefore suggested that this genetic material was replicated prior to mitosis. Improvements in auto-radiographic techniques, and especially the introduction of [^{3}H]-thymidine, quickly brought confirmation and then extensive ela-boration of the work of Howard and Pelc (1951).

Thymidine is a specific precursor of DNA and, when in-jected into animals, it is either incorporated into DNA or it is quickly (in less than an hour) broken down to nonutilizable pro-ducts. The nonincorporated thymidine and its derivatives are washed out by the common fixation procedures used in histology.

In this way, if thymidine is labeled with a radioactive isotope, usually [^{3}H] or [^{14}C], only the radioactivity incorporated into DNA remains in tissues after fixation. The result is that the nuclei of cells, which are synthesizing DNA at the time of exposure to [^{3}H] thymidine (± 30 minutes), are radioactive and can be identified by high resolution autoradiography (see monographs by Feinendegen 1967, by Rogers 1967, and by Baserga and Malamud 1969). In tissue culture thymidine is not broken down, but pulse-labeling can be easily obtained by exposing cells to [^{3}H] thymidine for 30 minutes and then changing back to a nonradioactive medium. In any case when eukaryotic cells are pulse-labeled with [^{3}H] thymidine, no labeled mitoses are found in autoradiographs of samples taken immediately after exposure to the radioactive precursor. However, after a few hours (depending on the cell population), labeled mitoses begin to appear and, if enough samples are taken at various intervals after a pulse exposure, one can draw a curve of percentage of labeled mitoses, as shown in Figure 1.1. The broken line in Figure 1.1 is the curve of percentage of labeled mitoses that would be obtained if all cells traversed the cell cycle asynchronously and at the same speed. However, even in clonal populations there is a considerable degree of variation among individual cells, and the resulting curve of percentage of labeled mitoses differs somewhat from the theoretical curve. The conclusions, however, remain the same. From the curve in Figure 1.1, it is possible to see that: (a) there is a discrete interval between completion of DNA synthesis and mitosis. This is the time required for the first labeled cells (which were cells synthesizing DNA at the time of exposure to [^{3}H] thymidine) to reach mitosis, and is called G_2 phase. (b) There is a period of DNA synthesis (S phase) roughly measured by the interval between the 50% points on the first ascending and descending limbs of the labeled mitoses curve; (c) mitosis (morphologically determined); and (d) a period between completion of mitosis and onset of DNA synthesis (G_1 phase). The cell cycle is defined as the interval between the midpoint of mitosis and the midpoint of the subsequent mitosis in one or both daughter cells and is schematically diagramed in Figure 1.2. The length of each phase of the cell cycle can be determined as shown in Figure 1.1, but it should be clearly understood at this point that the length of the cell cycle as a whole and of its component phases varies greatly from one cell population to another and among individual cells.

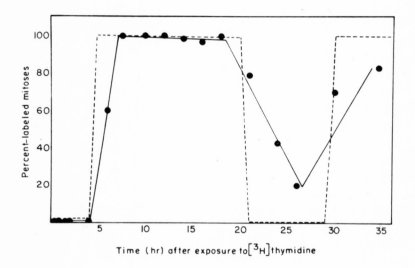

Time (hr) after exposure to [³H] thymidine

FIGURE 1.1   Percentage of labeled mitoses at various intervals after a 30-min exposure to [³H] thymidine. •—• actual autoradiographic values from WI-38 human diploid fibroblasts during exponential growth; — — — theoretical curve. The length of the cell cycle is given by the interval between the two 50% points on the first and second ascending limbs of the curve: 24.5 hr; the length of the S phase (DNA synthetic period) by the interval between the first ascending and the descending limb of the curve: 16.5 hr; the interval between completion of DNA synthesis and mitosis (G_2) is measured by a point 30 min after 0 time and the 50% point on the first ascending limb: 5 hr; since the duration of mitosis can be estimated at 1 hr, the duration of the interval between completion of mitosis and onset of DNA synthesis (G_1 phase) is obtained by default: 2 hr (for the derivation of these measurements, see Quastler and Sherman (1959) and Lamerton and Fry (1962).

CLASSIFICATION OF CELLS

The discovery of the cell cycle brought with it the suggestion that an orderly series of biochemical changes during interphase were a *conditio sine qua non* for mitosis itself. It also indicated that DNA was synthesized only in a discrete period of the interphase and, finally, it offered an explanation for the old observation of cytologists that the nuclear material was equally distributed between daughter cells at mitosis. By the time these studies were carried out, it was well known to molecular biologists that the amount of DNA per cell was constant for each species. The law of the constancy of DNA for each species had been put forward by Boivin, Vendrely, and Vendrely as far back as 1948 and, although the law suffers some exceptions, it still holds true as a generalization. If the amount of DNA per cell remains constant, it seems reasonable that a cell must duplicate its entire genetic material some time before mitosis.

Figure 1.2 represents the cell cycle of continuously dividing cells, corresponding to the vegetative intermitotics of Cowdry (1950). These are cell populations in which mitoses are commonly seen and which undergo the cyclic changes described above. Cells of this kind include the epithelial cells lining the crypts of the small intestine, the stem cells of the bone marrow, the cells of the basal layer of the epidermis, exponentially growing cells in culture, and others. The diagram of Figure 1.2 does not

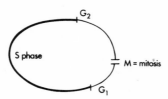

FIGURE 1.2   Diagram of the cell cycle of continuously dividing cells. After mitosis, there is a period (G_1 phase) during which the cell is preparing for DNA synthesis, but no DNA synthesis occurs. This G_1 phase is followed by the S phase, during which DNA is replicated. After completion of DNA replication, there is a third interval (G_2) during which the cell prepares for mitosis.

take into account cell populations in which mitoses are not seen
during the adult life of the animal, that is, the fixed postmitotic
cells of Cowdry (1950). The cell populations that Cowdry (1950)
classified as fixed postmitotics were more numerous then than
they are now. This is because with the use of more sensitive tools
it has become increasingly apparent that many cells previously
considered to be fixed postmitotics actually have the potential to
synthesize DNA and divide if an appropriate stimulus is applied.
These cell populations, which can be stimulated to synthesize
DNA and divide by an appropriate stimulus, will be discussed later.
Here, I will only remind the reader that even cells considered fixed
postmitotics through a longstanding reputation of over 100 years
(for instance, hen erythrocytes and neurons) can be stimulated to
synthesize DNA and divide under appropriate conditions. This is
not surprising since it is known that animal cells, even in the adult,
contain not only the same amount of DNA per cell characteristic
of each species but also the same amount of genetic information,
and, therefore, the necessary information for DNA synthesis and
cell division. The classic transplantation experiments of Briggs and
King (1952) have indicated that nuclei, in fact, contain all the
necessary information for the manyfold activities of the various
cell populations of the adult animal body. More recently, Laskey
and Gurdon (1970) have shown that when nuclei from adult
organs of *Xenopus laevis* are transplanted into enucleated eggs,
fully developed embryos can be obtained, indicating that nuclei of
adult somatic tissues contain the genetic information necessary for
the development of tadpoles and of many cell types. On the other
hand, no cytoplasmic heredity can be demonstrated with such
transplantation experiments (Gallien et al. 1973). The necessary
information for DNA synthesis and cell division, therefore, must
be present in practically all nucleated cells so that in the third
category of Cowdry (1950), the so-called *fixed postmitotic cells,*
we can now safely include only cells without a nucleus, or cells
that are partially enucleated, like the mature red blood cells of
mammalians, keratinizing cells of the epidermis, polymorphonuclear leukocytes, and a few others. Although these cells, which we
call nondividing cells, are extremely interesting for the study of

differentiation, they are of minor interest to the student of cell division and will not be further discussed in this monograph.

There remains the second category of cells, those classified by Cowdry (1950) as reverting postmitotics. These are cells, like hen erythrocytes and neurons mentioned above, which normally do not synthesize DNA nor divide but can be stimulated to do so by applying an appropriate stimulus. In the case of these two cells, the stimulus is fusion with another cell, like HeLa cells, which are continuously dividing cells. However, there are many other types of cells that ordinarily do not synthesize DNA nor divide but can be stimulated to do so. The oldest known example, of course, is the regenerating liver after partial hepatectomy. The ability of the liver to regenerate was first described by the ancient Greeks in the myth of Prometheus, chained to a mountain, whose liver was daily devoured by a vulture only to regenerate anew every night. Other populations of quiescent cells that can be stimulated to synthesize DNA and divide and that have been studied extensively include density-inhibited cell cultures stimulated by a change of medium (Todaro et al. 1965), phytohemagglutinin-stimulated lymphocytes (Cooper 1969), the isoproterenol-stimulated salivary gland (Barka 1965), and the estrogen-stimulated uterus (Hamilton 1968). These and other examples of stimulated cell proliferation (to be discussed in more detail in chapter 5) are all characterized by a lag between the application of the stimulus and the onset of DNA synthesis. The biochemical events occurring during the lag period will be the object of close scrutiny in later chapters. It suffices here to say that quiescent cells, in most cases, go through S before they divide (ie., G_0 comes before S), but in some instances quiescent cells (arrested in G_2) proceed directly to mitosis (Epifanova and Terskikh 1969).

With the addition of nondividing cells and of quiescent cells capable of DNA synthesis and cell division, the diagram of the cell cycle shown in Figure 1.2 must be modified to include these populations. The new diagram is shown in Figure 1.3. Continuously dividing cells correspond to Cowdry's vegetative intermitotics. Fixed postmitotics are now called nondividing cells and

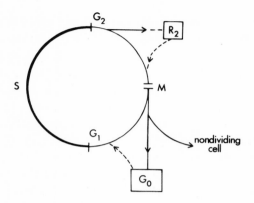

FIGURE 1.3   Cell populations and the cell cycle. Continuously dividing cells go around the cell cycle from one mitosis to the next. Nondividing cells have left the cycle and are destined to die without dividing again. G_0 cells are quiescent cells that can be stimulated to synthesize DNA and divide by an appropriate stimulus. R_2 cells are cells blocked in G_2, but can enter mitosis (without DNA replication) when stimulated.

reverting postmitotics are G_0 or R_2 cells (R_2 is the term proposed by Epifanova and Terskikh (1969) for cells arrested in G_2). In physiological conditions, cells may be arrested in G_1, G_2, or G_0, but not in S or mitosis. Cells that have begun S phase (or mitosis) proceed to complete DNA synthesis (or telophase) unless cell metabolism is grossly altered. Cells can stop in G_2 for very long times: one has only to think of tetraploid cells to realize that they are cells that have reached the G_2 phase but have not continued to mitosis. We shall discuss G_2-arrested cells in chapter 12, when considering the concepts of hypertrophy and hyperplasia. As to G_1-arrested and G_0 cells, a number of investigators have questioned the existence of G_0 cells and have suggested that G_0 cells are simply continuously dividing cells with a very long G_1 phase. While perfectly aware that this is, in the last analysis, a semantic problem, I would like to point out that if two cell populations can be distinguished from each other on the basis of some structural or functional characteristics, they ought to be recognized by different names. While a rose would smell as sweet by any other name, so would a carnation; yet, economy of language and the necessity of orderly interpersonal communication indicate the usefulness of using two different names. Similarly, if G_0 cells can be distinguished from G_1 cells, it would be easier to call them G_0 cells than to call them continuously dividing cells with a long G_1 period. The question is, therefore, "Can G_0 cells be distinguished by some structural or functional characteristic from G_1 cells"? There are now several reports in the literature indicating that G_0 cells can be distinguished from G_1 cells. The differences will be analyzed in chapter 11, after the reader has become familiar with the biochemical events occurring in G_1 and in G_0 cells stimulated to proliferate. For the moment, let the reader accept the statement that there are differences and that it is possible, therefore, to distinguish in the adult animal body three populations of cells: cells that continuously divide, nondividing cells, and quiescent cells that can be stimulated to divide by an appropriate stimulus.

THE THREE PARAMETERS OF
THE POPULATION EXPLOSION

The next important step in our story is to recognize that the classification of cells into three types applies to populations of different cells as well as to similar cells within a homogeneous clonal population. Not only cultured cells (Martin et al. 1974) but many tissues of the adult animal consist of a mixture of similar cells that includes continuously dividing cells, quiescent cells that occasionally go back to the cell cycle, and nondividing cells. For instance, in certain tumors there are cells that divide continuously, other cells that do not participate in the proliferating process but may be brought back to the cell cycle by an immunological stimulus, and dying cells (De Cosse and Gelfant 1968). If one now looks again at the diagram in Figure 1.3, one can easily understand how the growth of a cell population is regulated by three parameters, namely: (a) the length of the cell cycle, (b) the fraction of nondividing cells, and (c) the fraction of G_0 cells, that is, cells momentarily out of the cell cycle but capable of returning to the cycle

under appropriate circumstances. (Cells can also grow in size, as
we shall see in chapter 12, but for the moment we are only concerned with growth in the number of cells). The first and third
parameters determine the number of new cells produced per unit
time, while the second parameter influences the rate of cell death.
When the number of cells produced equals the number of cells
that die, the cell population remains constant in number and is
said to be in a steady state (see Lamerton and Fry 1962, passim).
When the number of cells produced per unit time exceeds the
number of dying cells, the cell population increases in number,
that is, grows. This is, in fact, what happens in the developing embryo and newborn animal where persistent cell division with very
little cell loss brings about a continuous increase in the number of
cells. Indeed, it does not take a profound observer to realize that
cell division is an important factor in growth, since animals derive
from a single cell, the fertilized egg. The number of cells in an
adult animal can be estimated somewhat roughly by remembering
that in mammalian cells the content of DNA per cell is 7×10^{-12} g.
A mouse, 22-25 g in weight, contains a total of 20 mg of DNA,
which means 3×10^9 cells. If we assume that the number of cells
per gram of tissue is about the same in human as in mouse tissues,
one can calculate that in a 70-kg man there are roughly 10^{13} cells.

If growth is regulated by the above-mentioned three
parameters, an increase in the number of cells in a given cell population may be accomplished by one of four mechanisms: (a) a
shortening of the cell cycle of continuously dividing cells, (b) an
increase in the fraction of dividing cells, that is, an increase in the
growth fraction, with recruiting of G_0 cells into the cell cycle, (c)
a decrease in the rate of cell loss, and (d) a combination of the
above. The importance of these mechanisms in the growth of normal tissues has been known to investigators for a number of years
(see Lamerton and Fry 1962, passim). It is also known that the
growth of tumors (either in experimental animals or man) also depends on these parameters, and, in fact, shortening of the cell
cycle, increase in the growth fraction, and a decrease in the rate of
cell loss have all been described in tumor cell populations. The
relative importance of these parameters has been analyzed in detail
by Norrby (1970) in populations of cells in culture, that is, in a

closed system where the number of cells in each stage could be measured with accuracy. Norrby (1970) compared diploid human normal fetal cells and human fetal cells transformed by infection with the DNA oncogenic virus SV-40. Transformed cells (comparable in some respects to tumor cells) grew to a higher density than did their normal counterparts. The ability of transformed cells to reach a higher saturation density than normal cells is firmly established in the literature (Kruse et al. 1969, Ponten 1971). In Norrby's case, under the same nutritional conditions, normal fetal cell lines grew to a density of 9-16 $\times$ 10^4 cells per square centimeter, whereas SV-40 transformed fetal cells grew to a density of 15-44 $\times$ 10^4 cells per square centimeter. Yet, the length of the cell cycle in these two cell populations was substantially the same, ie., 13.5 hours in normal cells and 13.6 hours in SV-40 transformed cells. The death rate, however, was higher in normal cells than in transformed cells. For instance, the death index (that is, the effective death rate in percent of the effective birth rate) was 19.6% in normal cells and only 7.5% in transformed cells. In these cultures the growth fraction was unity or near unity in most cases, but, because of the decreased cell loss, the effective growth rate (expressed in cells per hour) was 59.7 in normal cells and 67.8 in transformed cells.

TUMOR GROWTH

These results, which show that transformed cells do not have a shorter cell cycle than their normal counterparts, confirmed the report by Baserga and Kisieleski (1962) that the cell cycle of continuously dividing normal cells of mice can be shorter than the cell cycle of some of the fastest growing mouse tumors. Their findings indicated that the growth of tumors in vivo does not necessarily depend on an increased speed of cellular proliferation, that is, on a shortening of the cell cycle, but that it may depend on other factors as, for instance, the growth fraction and the rate of cell loss. Their results have been confirmed by numerous data subsequently gathered in experimental animals and in man. Some illustrative examples of cell cycle times are given in Table 1.1. A cursory glance at this table shows that a shortening of the cell cycle is not necessary for producing the increase in total number of cells observed in tumors. An increase in growth fraction has been shown to be operative in some cases (see the data of Clarkson et al. 1965, and those collected by Gavosto and Pileri 1971), but the decreased rate of cell loss is also important. Although the rate of cell loss cannot be calculated with precision in human tumors, it has been shown to be decreased in some tumors in experimental animals (Steel et al. 1966). The conclusion from these data is that cell division may occur in a variety of tissues but that cell multiplication occurs only in the embryo, in certain tissues of the growing animal, and in some disturbances of growth, including cancer. This is an important concept to keep in mind, namely, that cell division can occur in nongrowing cell populations at the same speed or even faster than in growing tissues. Therefore, when we wish to know the factors that control the size of a cell population, we have to ask ourselves not only what are the factors that control the flow of cells through the cell cycle but also what are the factors that influence the recruiting of G_0 cells into the cell cycle and the rate of cell loss. We shall omit the latter from further discussion in this monograph (which is concerned with division and multiplication, but not with subtraction) and concentrate, instead, on factors that control cell division and the recruiting of G_0 cells into the cell cycle. The rest of the monograph will then be devoted to the questions, "What is the molecular basis for the control of cellular proliferation in continuously dividing cells and in G_0 cells stimulated to proliferate"?

A glance at Figure 1.3 seems to indicate that if we wish to understand the mechanism that controls cellular proliferation, we ought to understand first the mechanism that controls DNA synthesis. This is because in the great majority of cases DNA synthesis in mammalian cells is followed at a short interval by cell division, and also because (and again in the great majority of cases) when G_0 cells are stimulated to proliferate they first enter DNA synthesis and then divide. There are, of course, a number of exceptions to this rule (G_2-arrested cells, mentioned above and to be

TABLE 1.1   Selected Cell Cycle Times (Tc) of Some Normal Tissues and Tumors

Tissue	Tc (hr)	Tissue	Tc (hr)
Mouse			
Duodenal crypt cells[a]	10.3	Ehrlich ascites tumor[a]	36
Mammary gland, alveoli[a]	71	Transplantable fibrosarcoma[a]	17.5
Antibody-forming cells[a]	9	C3H mammary tumor[a]	3.5 days
Embryo ependymal cells[a]	11		
Rat			
Liver cells[a]	47.5	Internal enamel epithelium[a]	27.3
Spleen germinal centers[a]	13.4	Yoshida ascites hepatoma[a]	45
Man			
Colon, crypt cells[a]	39	Basal cell carcinoma of skin[a]	36
Rectum, crypt cells[a]	48	Bronchus, carcinoma[b]	196-260
Bronchus, epithelial cells[b]	220	Carcinoma stomach[a]	72
Trachea, epithelial cells[b]	448	Acute myeloblastic	
Carcinoma endometrium[a]	110	leukemia[a]	80-84
Lymphosarcoma[a]	91	Chronic myeloid leukemia[a]	120
Tissue cultures			
HeLa cells[a]	21	WI-38 human diploid	
Glioma cells[c]	32	fibroblasts[a]	24.5
L-mouse cells[a]	23	Glia-like cells (diploid)[c]	22

[a]*Data reported by several investigators and collected by Baserga and Malamud (1969), by Lipkin (1971), and by Gavosto and Pileri (1971).*
[b]*From Fabrikant (1970).*
[c]*From Ponten et al. (1969) and Westermark (1973).*

discussed in a later chapter). For the moment let us simply say that, with few exceptions DNA synthesis is followed at a short interval by mitosis. Figure 1.3 also shows that cells synthesizing DNA and dividing may originate from two different sources: continuously dividing cells and G_0 cells stimulated to proliferate. The biochemical processes occurring during the S phase, G_2, or mitosis are substantially the same in the two groups of cells and can be discussed as common entities. We shall therefore, in the next few chapters, discuss in detail the biochemistry of S, G_2, and mitosis, three phases of the cell cycle that are common to continuously dividing cells and to G_0 cells stimulated to proliferate. We shall then consider separately the biochemistry of the G_1 phase and the prereplicative phase of G_0 cells, that is, the sequences of biochemical events that precede and presumably control the onset of DNA synthesis, respectively, in continuously dividing cells and in stimulated G_0 cells. The second half of the monograph will be devoted to the intimate molecular mechanisms that trigger the sequence of biochemical events eventually leading to DNA synthesis and cell division. Finally, in the last two chapters we shall try to apply what has been learned about the molecular basis of cell proliferation to the explanation of some disturbances of growth, including cancer.

Before proceeding, remember once more that the entire monograph deals only with those cellular processes strictly connected with the flow of cells through the cell cycle. Energy production, macromolecular synthesis and degradation, secretion, motility, and all the various metabolic activities which occur in cycling as well as in noncycling cells will not be considered here unless they specifically relate to the cell cycle traverse or the prereplicative phase of stimulated G_0 cells.

Again, this monograph is intended to deal with mammalian cells only and work on lower animals and prokaryotes will be discussed only when needed to illustrate or better explain a given point. For those interested in the biochemistry of the cell cycle of lower animals or bacteria, the excellent monograph by Mitchison (1971) and two other reviews, one by Lark (1969) on bacteria and one by Hartwell et al. (1974) on yeasts are recommended.

REFERENCES

Avery, O. T., MacLeod, C. M., and McCarty, M. (1944) *J. Exp. Med. 79*: 137-158.

Barka, T. (1965). *Exp. Cell Res. 39*: 355-364.

Baserga, R. and Kisieleski, W. E. (1962). *J. Natl. Cancer Inst. 28*: 331-339.

Baserga, R. and Malamud, D. (1969). *Autoradiography; Techniques and Application.* Harper and Row, New York.

Boivin, A., Vendrely, R., and Vendrely, C. (1948). *Compt. Rend. 226*: 1061-1063.

Briggs, R. and King, T. J. (1952). *Proc. Natl. Acad. Sci. 38*: 455-463.

Clarkson, B., Ota, K., Ohkita, T., and O'Connor, A. (1965). *Cancer 18*: 1189-1213.

Cooper, H. L. (1969). In *Biochemistry of Cell Division*, R. Baserga (Ed.) C. C. Thomas, Springfield, Illinois, pp. 91-112.

Cowdry, E. V. (1950). *Textbook of Histology.* Lea and Febiger, Philadelphia.

DeCosse, J. J. and Gelfant, S. (1968). *Science 162*: 698-699.

Epifanova, O. I. and Terskikh, V. V. (1969). *Cell Tissue Kinet. 2*: 75-93.

Fabrikant, J. I. (1970). *Br. J. Cancer 24*: 122-127.

Feinendegen, L. E. (1967). *Tritium-labeled Molecules in Biology and Medicine.* Academic Press, New York.

Gallien, C., Aimar, C., and Guillet, F. (1973). *Develop. Biol. 33*: 154-170.

Gavosto, F. and Pileri, A. (1971). In *The Cell Cycle and Cancer,* R. Baserga (Ed.). Dekker, New York, pp. 99-128.

Hamilton, T. H. (1968). *Science 161*: 649-661.

Hartwell, L. H., Culotti, J., Pringle, J. R., and Reid, B. J. (1974). *Science 183*: 46-51.

Hershey, A. D. and Chase, M. (1952). *J. Gen. Physiol. 36*: 39-56.

Howard, A. and Pelc, S. R. (1951). *Exp. Cell Res. 2*: 178-187.

Kruse, P. F. Jr., Whittle, W., and Miedema, E. (1969). *J. Cell Biol. 42*: 113-121.

Lamerton, L. F. and Fry, R. J. M. (Eds.) (1962). *Cell Proliferation.* Blackwell, Oxford.

Lark, K. G. (1969). *Ann. Rev. Biochem. 38*: 569-604.

Laskey, R. A. and Gurdon, J. B. (1970). *Nature 288*: 1332-1334.

Lipkin, M. (1971). In *The Cell Cycle and Cancer,* R. Baserga, (Ed.). Dekker, New York, pp. 6-26.

Martin, G. M., Sprague, C. A., Norwood, T. H., and Pendergrass, W. R. (1974). *Am. J. Pathol. 74*: 137-154.

Mayzel, W. (1875). *Zbl. Med. Wiss. 13*: 849-852.

Mitchison, J. M. (1971). *The Biology of the Cell Cycle.* Cambridge University Press, London.

Norrby, K. (1970). *Acta Pathol. Microbiol. Scand. 78 (suppl. 214)*: 3-49.

Ponten, J. (1971). *Spontaneous and Virus Induced Transformation in Cell Culture.* Springer-Verlag, New York, p. 253.

Ponten, J., Westermark, B., and Hugosson, R. (1969). *Exp. Cell Res. 58*: 393-400.

Quastler, H. and Sherman, F. G. (1959). *Exp. Cell Res. 17*: 420-438.

Rogers, A. W. (1967). *Techniques of Autoradiography.* Elsevier, Amsterdam.

Rusconi, M. (1826). Sur le Developpement de la Grenouille commune depuis le Moment de sa Naissance jusqu'a son Etat parfait. Milan.

Steel, G. G., Adams, K., and Barrett, J. C. (1966). *Br. J. Cancer 20*: 784-800.

Todaro, G. J., Lazar, G. K., and Green, H. (1965). *J. Cell. Comp. Physiol. 66*: 325-334.

Westermark, B. (1973). *Int. J. Cancer 12*: 438-451.

TWO

S PHASE

DEFINITION OF S PHASE

The main event during the S phase is the replication of genetic material, that is, DNA, histones, and nonhistone chromosomal proteins. As stated by Gerald Mueller (1971): "The spectacular achievement of the S phase is that its active and inactive chromatin are replicated and distributed with precision to the daughter chromosomes assuring both phenotypic and genetic continuity." And, just as in the cell cycle, there is an orderly sequence of biochemical changes that regulate the flow of cells from one phase to the next, similarly the progression of cells from the beginning to the end of S is controlled by a series of steps that eventually result in the complete replication of chromosomal components.

SYNCHRONIZATION OF CELLS

To study these steps if is often necessary to use a methodology which has been extremely valuable in increasing our knowledge of the biochemical events occuring in various phases of the cell cycle, ie., the synchronization of cell populations in culture. The numerous methods for synchronizing cells in vitro (see

reviews by Frindel and Tubiana 1971 and by Nias and Fox 1971)
can be conveniently divided into two large groups: (a) physical
methods, and (b) chemical methods (to which one can always add
a third possibility, ie., a combination of both). Physical methods
include mitotic selection, which is based on the fact that mammalian cells grown in monolayer cultures are less firmly attached
to the growing surface during mitosis and can be selectively detached by gently agitating the growth vessel (Terasima and Tolmach 1963). The mitotic selection technique gives a small yield of
cells but a high degree of synchronization and disturbs the vital
processes of the cell very little. Unfortunately, this method can be
applied only to cells growing in monolayer cultures. Among other
physical methods, gradient techniques and volume selection are of
some interest but give a moderate degree of synchronization (Nias
and Fox 1971). The gradient method, however, may be somewhat
useful in separating G_1, S, and G_2 growing in suspension cultures,
such as human lymphoid cells (Everson et al. 1973). A great number of chemical methods have been used for synchronizing cells in
culture, including high concentrations of thymidine in the growth
medium (eg., 2 mM or more), hydroxyurea, and several other compounds discussed in detail in the two references given above. All of
these chemical methods produce, to some extent, what has been
called *unbalanced growth* and, although they have been used extensively, the results obtained with these methods are open to a
considerable amount of criticism (Studzinski and Lambert 1969).
However, the abnormal cellular composition caused by excess
thymidine was found to revert to control levels by the time of the
first mitosis (Lambert and Studzinski 1969). It is therefore possible to use a combination of methods which could result in normal
function and a good yield, ie., a double-thymidine block of cells in
suspension, followed by plating at the time of release of the
second block, and selective mitotic detachment several hours later
(Stein and Borun 1972).

Another method for synchronizing cells in suspension
culture, which has merit, is the isoleucine-deprivation technique.
With this procedure, cells are arrested in early G_1 (or G_0) by growing them in isoleucine-deficient medium, from which they can be

induced to traverse the cell cycle again by simply adding isoleucine (Ley and Tobey 1970). Each method has its advantages and its shortcomings. Suffice it to say here that by appropriate manipulations, cultured cells can by synchronized in any phase of the cell cycle with, at most, only 10% of the cell population being out of phase. Matters are different, though, if one wishes a precise degree of synchrony, for instance, all cells ± 10 minutes at the same point in the cycle. Some published methods are more impressive than others, because the charts are drawn with short abscissae and tall ordinates, but the truth of the matter is that even with mitotic de-teachment, the entrance of synchronized cells into S is spread over a period of hours.

DNA SYNTHESIS: FACTORS REQUIRED

Returning to our main topic, let us look at those cell cycle-related events during S and begin with DNA, the synthesis of which is necessary for the progression of cells from the G_1/S boundary to the S/G_2 boundary. Since I presume that the reader is already familiar with the fundamental principles of DNA synthesis in bacteria, I will limit myself here to a brief description of the main factors required that are relevant to our discussion. The isolation by DeLucia and Cairns (1969) of a mutant of *Escherichia coli* (W3110 Thy-pol A), which possesses only a few percent of the classic Kornberg DNA polymerase activity when assayed in vitro but which is, nevertheless, able to replicate its DNA normally, has indicated that the actual mechanism of DNA replication does not involve the Kornberg polymerase. In fact, evidence indicates that the Kornberg polymerase, (hereafter called *DNA polymerase I*) may be required for DNA repair but not for DNA replication (although it may replace other enzymes in the incorporation of Okazaki fragments into longer DNA chains). The true DNA replicase (hereafter called *DNA polymerase III*) has been identified in bacteria by using temperature-sensitive mutants (Gefter et al. 1971). The general consensus, now, is that DNA replication in *E. coli* requires DNA polymerase III, that its role is not clear but it is

probably necessary for DNA elongation, that DNA polymerase I is
involved in DNA repair (see reviews by Moses et al. 1972 and
Hirota et al. 1972), and that DNA polymerase II may participate
in chain elongation (Tait and Smith 1974). A mammalian DNA
polymerase involved in DNA replication has been tentatively identified in HeLa cell nuclei by Friedman (1970). It appears from the
studies of Mueller and coworkers (1971) and of Friedman (1970)
that, while DNA polymerase I is found largely in the cytosol of
HeLa cells lysed in aqueous media, the true DNA replicase is essentially a nuclear enzyme with slightly different properties from
DNA polymerase I. Interestingly enough, DNA polymerase I activity is roughly constant throughout the cell cycle of continuously
dividing mammalian cells, whereas DNA polymerase III activity increases just before the onset of DNA synthesis and decreases again
when cells enter the G_2 phase. Essentially similar results have been
reported by Spadari and Weissbach (1974) who, however, use a
different terminology: R-DNA polymerase for the polymerase that
parallels DNA synthesis and D-DNA polymerase II for the cytoplasmic enzyme, the activity of which reaches a maximum after
DNA synthesis has ceased.

The ability of isolated nuclei to synthesize DNA is
highly dependent on soluble protein factors from the cell lysate,
which are essential for the progression of DNA synthesis (see review by Mueller 1971). In this respect, it is worthwhile to remember that when HeLa cells in G_1 are fused with HeLa cells in S
phase, DNA synthesis is promptly induced in the G_1 nuclei (Rao
and Johnson 1970). The presence of cytoplasmic factors, though,
may be a necessary but not sufficient prerequisite, since in multi-
nucleated ovarian cancer cells, DNA synthesis in the various nuclei
is often asynchronous (Sheehy et al. 1974). Alternatively, these
two seemingly contradictory findings could be reconciled by the
elegant experiments of Gonzalez-Fernandez et al. (1971) on poly-
nucleated cells of root meristems of *Albium cepa*, showing that all
nuclei of a given cell enter S phase synchronously but leave it
asynchronously.

In mammalian cells, as in bacteria, it appears that DNA
is synthesized in short segments, the so-called *Okazaki fragments*

(Sato et al. 1970), which, on becoming contiguous, are ligated into longer chains by another enzyme, polynucleotide ligase. Recent evidence in phages and bacteria also indicates that RNA polymerase and some kinds of RNA chains are a necessary requirement for DNA synthesis (Wickner et al. 1972), as if a macromolecular product of RNA polymerase (possibly a short RNA chain) were a primer for the initiation of DNA synthesis. In fact, according to Lark (1972), RNA is directly involved as part of the DNA replication fork in *E. coli*. Some evidence that newly synthesized short RNA chains are covalently bound to nascent DNA and serve as primers for DNA replication has also been found in mammalian cells (Sato et al. 1972, Nicolini and Baserga 1974). These findings are probably related to the results reported several years ago by Feinendegen et al. (1961) in HeLa cells, results which at that time seemed rather puzzling. These authors found that a fraction of RNA was involved in providing precursors for subsequent DNA replication and, although their data were purely of a kinetic nature, they still stand as a suitable model for determining the role of RNA fragments in the initiation of DNA synthesis in mammalian cells.

In addition to DNA polymerase III, polynucleotide ligase, an RNA primer, and the DNA template, a number of other enzymes and the deoxynucleotide triphosphates are involved in DNA replication. As it becomes a DNA topic, there is a highly repetitive literature on the pool size of deoxynucleotide precursors and on the concentration of various enzymes connected with the synthesis and phosphorylation of these precursors in quiescent and proliferating cells. This is because, for a while, a number of investigators firmly believed that the concentration of these precursors and/or enzymes (including DNA polymerase), played a decisive role in the control of DNA synthesis in bacteria and in mammalian cells. This idea, which reached its peak of popularity about 10 to 15 years ago, still has a lot of followers. Indeed, when an investigator, whether wholly inexperienced (novice) or experienced, but in another field (neophyte), decides to enter the field of cellular proliferation, chances are that one of his first papers will be dealing with the concentration of certain deoxynucleotides or enzymes, such as thymidine kinase, thymidylate synthetase, and so forth, and their role in the control of DNA synthesis. As it happens in such cases, the neophyte is often more sanguine about it than the novice. The mistake is made easy by the fact that DNA synthesis in vitro can be promptly stopped by subtracting from the reaction mixture one of the deoxynucleotide precursors or one of the required enzymes. The same effect can be obtained in vivo with appropriate inhibitors. However, while deoxynucleotide precursors and the enzymes that synthesize and phosphorylate them are a necessary requirement for DNA synthesis, the decisional control of DNA replication lies, as we shall see in the next chapters, further back. By the time a cell enters DNA synthesis, a number of critical decisions have already been made and are the critical steps that ought to be considered the real controlling factors in DNA synthesis. It is not surprising, then, that the concentration of deoxynucleotides and of a variety of related enzymes does not follow closely the cell cycle (see review by Baserga 1968). Thus, while the activity of certain enzymes, such as thymidine kinase, and the concentration of deoxynucleotides do increase during the S phase, they remain elevated during G_2 and mitosis when DNA synthesis has completely ceased (Bray and Brent 1972). In stimulated 3T3 cells, coincidentally with the onset of DNA synthesis, there is an increase in the uptake of thymidine and deoxycitidine, but not of purine deoxynucleosides or orthophosphate (Cunningham and Remo 1973). Similarly, there is no correlation between the size of the deoxyribonucleotide pool and the onset of DNA synthesis in explanted rabbit kidney cells (Adams et al. 1966). Among enzymes related to DNA synthesis, ribonucleotide reductase is a good example: in regenerating liver after partial hepatectomy it begins to increase at 24 hours, reaching a maximum at 50 hours (Larsson1969), while DNA synthesis increases at 18 hours, peaks at 20, and by 48 hours it is back almost to control levels (Grisham 1962). Even worse is the case of polynucleotide ligase, the increase in activity of which, in phytohemagglutinin-stimulated lymphocytes, is delayed 1 day with respect to the increase in DNA synthesis (Pedrini et al. 1972). However, the best demonstration of the role of the DNA-synthesizing machinery in the control of DNA replication can be found in the experiments of Gurdon et al. (1969) who injected DNA into unfertilized frogs' eggs. The foreign DNA was promptly replicated, indicating that the egg cytoplasm contained, ready to go, the whole DNA-synthesizing machinery. One could say that deoxynucleotides and related enzymes are like the bricks and the masons necessary to build a home. Undoubtedly one cannot build a brick home without masons and bricks, but it is obvious that the decision to build the home is made elsewhere.

In the category of molecules important for DNA replication we can probably include a specific protein (or class of proteins) necessary for the initiation of DNA synthesis in each replicon. A DNA-binding protein, absent from cells in which DNA synthesis is specifically blocked, has been reported in *E. coli* by Masker and Eberle (1971) and may be analogous to the DNA "melting protein" described by Alberts et al. (1968). This protein is thought to have a role at the replication fork (see review by von Hippel and McGhee 1972). Very little, however, is known about the nature of these initiator proteins.

ASYNCHRONOUS REPLICATION OF CHROMOSOMES

It has been known for some time that DNA replication in chromosomes is a multifocal phenomenon along the length of the various chromosomes (Stubblefield and Mueller 1962) and that a definite temporal order exists for the replication of different DNA units of a cell nucleus. For instance, the genes coding for ribosomal RNA in Chinese hamster cells are replicated in the first half of the S phase (Stambrook 1974); so is the viral genome that is an integral part of the DNA of human lymphoblastoid cells latently infected with the Epstein-Barr herpesvirus (Hampar et al. 1974). In general DNA that is replicated in the early S phase is relatively rich in guanine and cytosine (G + C-rich DNA), while late replicating DNA is relatively A + T-rich. Other observations have indicated that heterochromatin is synthesized late in the S phase, but according to later investigations there is no correlation between the late replication of heterochromatin and the synthesis of A + T-rich DNA toward the end of the replication (Bostok and

Prescott 1971). However, multiple replication units (so-called *replicons*) of 10 to 100 μm in length (40 to 400 μm for Stubblefield 1973) are clearly a feature of DNA replication in higher organisms (Painter and Rasmussen 1964) and, in fact, these replicons can be separated from bulk DNA as a replication complex containing nascent cellular DNA (Pearson and Hanawalt 1971). In Chinese hamster cells, replicons are arranged in early and late replicating clusters, and in each cluster individual replicons replicate at different times (Hori and Lark 1973, Hand and Tamm 1974). Puromycin inhibits the initiation of DNA replication in replicons (which, in Chinese hamster cells, are units ranging in length from 20 to 70 μm and replicating at a rate of 1 μm/min) but does not inhibit chain elongation in a replicon which has already begun DNA synthesis at the time the drug is added (Hori and Lark 1973). In *E. coli* there is clear evidence that chromosome replication is bidirectional (Prescott and Kuempel 1972), but in mammalian cells the evidence is still circumstantial. Replicons can be translated, at the cytological level, into the previously mentioned observation by Stubblefield and Mueller (1962) that DNA replication in chromosomes is a multifocal phenomenon (see also Taylor 1960 and Painter 1961). A typical example is given by the χ chromosome of female cells. One of the χ chromosomes begins replication later in S phase and completes replication after all other chromosomes have completed DNA synthesis (Morishima et al. 1962, Moorhead and Defendi 1963). For instance, in human fibroblasts, the inactive χ chromosome does not begin DNA replication until 2.5 hours after onset of DNA synthesis and continues replication for 1.6 hours after most DNA has ceased replication (Comings 1967). Finally, it should be mentioned that in mammalian cells, replication sites for chromosomal DNA occur throughout the nucleus and are not preferentially associated with the nuclear envelope (Fakan et al. 1972, Huberman et al. 1973).

CONCOMITANT EVENTS TO DNA REPLICATION

Several other events accompany DNA synthesis in the nucleus and are related either directly to it or to the flow of cells through the cell cycle. For instance, in diploid cells the synthesis of microtubular proteins begins at mid S, eventually to continue throughout G_2 (Forrest and Klevecz 1972), and centrioles present in G_1 commence replication at about the same time that DNA synthesis begins (Robbins et al. 1968). In mouse L cells, poly ADP-ribose is synthesized in two short-lived bursts during S (Colyer et al. 1973).

During the S phase, chromosomal proteins are replicated together with DNA. Chromosomal proteins (which we will study in more detail in chapter 7), can be divided into two large groups, histones (basic proteins that do not contain tryptophan) and non-histone chromosomal proteins (generally acidic, containing trypto-phan and rich in glutamic and aspartic acids). Histones, as shown in the classic experiments of Borun et al. (1967), are synthesized during the S phase. While a slight turnover of F_1 histone may be taking place in other phases of the cell cycle (Gurley and Hardin 1970), it is now generally agreed that the amount of histones is doubled during the S phase (Gurley and Hardin 1968) simultaneously with the replication of DNA, and that the bulk of these proteins are essentially conserved through successive cell generations (Hancock 1969). Histones are synthesized in the cytoplasm and are then transferred to the nucleus where they bind to DNA, newly synthesized histones binding to newly synthesized DNA (Tsanev and Russev 1974). When histone synthesis is inhibited, as for instance with cycloheximide or other inhibitors of protein synthesis, the synthesis of DNA ceases after a few minutes. This is quite reasonable. If histones are, as it is generally assumed, aspecific repressors of DNA transcription, it is of the utmost importance that they be replicated simultaneously with DNA. If the newly synthesized DNA were not promptly repressed by newly synthe-sized histones, it could be transcribed, with some rather weird con-sequences for the cell. Conversely, when DNA synthesis is in-hibited, as for instance by hydroxyurea, the synthesis of histones promptly ceases.

Histones can also be modified by acetylation, phosphor-ylation, or methylation, a phenomenon that will be dealt with in detail in a later chapter. One should mention here that histone F_1, which is dephosphorylated during G_1, is phosphorylated again when DNA replication begins, until eventually over 90% of all histone F_1 molecules are converted into two phosphorylated forms (Marks et al. 1973).

Also synthesized during the S phase are nonhistone chromosomal proteins. An essential component of chromatin structure, nonhistone chromosomal proteins, at variance with histones, are synthesized at the same rate in all phases of the cell cycle (Stein and Baserga 1970, Cross 1972) and their synthesis is not inhibited when DNA synthesis is inhibited by hydroxyurea (Zampetti-Bosseler et al. 1969). In addition, nonhistone chromosomal proteins synthesized during the S phase are indistinguishable by gel electrophoresis from nonhistone chromosomal proteins synthesized in other phases of the cell cycle (except G_0 cells, as we shall see later).

The synthesis of RNA also continues during the S phase. A constant rate of RNA synthesis during S phase has been thought to be unlikely becuase DNA transcription and replication cannot occur simultaneously. That RNA synthesis is, in fact, suppressed during DNA replication has been demonstrated by the elegant experiments of Prescott (1962) with cultures of Euplotes in which DNA synthesis occurs as a double wave propagating from the tips to the center of the macronucleus. Synthesis of RNA can be observed autoradiographically over the entire nucleus, except in correspondence of the two bands of DNA synthesis where RNA synthesis is totally absent. However, in mammalian cells DNA synthesis is markedly asynchronous, the asynchrony affecting not only individual chromosomes but also different segments in each chromosome. Considering that the molecular weight of mammalian DNA is approximately the same as that of *E. coli* DNA and knowing the speed with which deoxynucleotides can be polymerized into DNA, one can quickly calculate that the entire replication of a DNA molecule having a molecular weight of 10^9 daltons should require only 20-30 minutes. The fact that the mammalian cell nucleus takes from 8-20 hours to replicate DNA (see Table 2.1) indicates that different molecules of DNA (replicons?) are replicated at different times and that at any given moment in the S phase

TABLE 2.1   Duration of S Phase in Representative Cells

Cell type	Duration of S (hr)	Reference
Mouse		
embryo primitive ependymal cells	5.5	Atlas and Bond (1965)
esophageal epithelium	8.5	Blenkinsopp (1969)
duodenal epithelial cells	7.9	Lesher et al. (1961)
mammary gland, normal alveoli		
in intact females	21.7	Bresciani (1965)
in estrogen-treated females	9.2	Bresciani (1965)
Rat		
cells of splenic germinal centers	4.5	Fliedner et al. (1964)
Man		
epithelian cells of colon	14.0	Lipkin et al. (1962)
trachea	13.0	Fabrikant (1970)
bronchus	11.3	Fabrikant (1970)
bronchus carcinoma	21-23	Fabrikant (1970)
esophageal carcinoma	22-25	Fabrikant (1970)
erythropoietic cells	11-13	Stryckmans et al. (1966)
basal cell carcinoma of skin	19.0	Malaise et al. (1967)
metastatic carcinoma of colon	20.0	Clarkson et al. (1965)
Human diploid cells in culture	7.5	Defendi and Manson (1963)
L-mouse cells	12.2	Cleaver (1965)
HeLa S_3 cells	9.5	Terasima and Tolmach (1963)

only about 5%-15% of the DNA is being replicated. Under these circumstances it is not surprising that a decrease in the rate of RNA synthesis in mammalian cells during the S phase is not detectable by conventional laboratory methods. However, at least in *Physarum polycephalum*, RNA synthesized during the S phase contains sequences not present in RNA synthesized during G_2 (Fouquet and Braun 1974).

In conclusion, despite and perhaps because of the complexities of chromosomal replication, the S phase cell is a cell almost exclusively geared to chromatin replication and remarkably lacking in independence. It is a cell without a life of its own, a cell that has been both programmed (by a decision taken a few hours before) and committed (to mitosis, a few hours later). Before looking at the events preceding the onset of DNA synthesis, let us follow the S cell to its logical moira, mitosis.

REFERENCES

Adams, R. L. P., Abrams, R., and Lieberman, I. (1966). *J. Biol. Chem. 241:* 903-905.

Alberts, B. M., Amodio, F. J., Jenkins, M., Gutman, E. D., and Ferris, F. L. (1968). *Cold Spring Harbor Symp. Quant. Biol.* 33:289-305.

Atlas, M. and Bond, V. P. (1965). *J. Cell Biol. 26:* 19-24.

Baserga, R. (1968). *Cell Tissue Kinet. 1:* 167-191.

Blenkinsopp, W. K. (1969). *J. Cell Sci. 5:* 393-401.

Borun, T. W., Scharff, M. D., and Robbins, E. (1967). *Proc. Natl. Acad. Sci. 58:* 1977-1983.

Bostok, C. J. and Prescott, D. M. (1971). *J. Molec. Biol. 60:* 151-162.

Bray, G. and Brent, T. P. (1972). *Biochim. Biophys. Acta. 269:* 184-191.

Bresciani, F. (1965). In *Cellular Radiation Biology*, M. D. Anderson Symp., Williams and Wilkins, Baltimore, pp. 547-557.

Clarkson, B., Ota, K., Ohkita, T., and O'Connor, A. (1965). *Cancer 18:* 1189-1213.

Cleaver, J. E. (1965). *Exp. Cell Res. 39:* 697-700.

Colyer, R. A., Burdette, K. E., and Kidwell, W. R. (1973). *Biochem. Biophys. Res. Comm. 53:* 960-966.

Comings, D. E. (1967). *Cytogenetics 6:* 20-37.

Cross, M. L. (1972). *Biochem. J. 128:* 1213-1219.

Cunningham, D. D. and Remo, R. A. (1973). *J. Biol. Chem. 248:* 6282-6288.

Defendi, V. and Manson, L. A. (1963). *Nature 198:* 359-361.

De Lucia, P. and Cairns, J. (1969). *Nature 224:* 1164-1166.

Everson, L. K., Buell, D. N., and Rogentine, G. N. Jr. (1973). *J. Exp. Med. 137:* 343-358.

Fabrikant, J. I. (1970). *Br. J. Cancer 24:* 122-127.

Fakan, S., Turner, G. N., Pagano, J. S., and Hancock, R. (1972). *Proc. Natl. Acad. Sci. 69:* 2300-2305.

Feinendegen, L. E., Bond, V. P., and Hughes, W. L. (1961). *Exp. Cell Res. 25:* 627-647.

Fliedner, T. M., Kesse, M., Cronkite, E. P., and Robertson, J. S. (1964). *Ann. N.Y. Acad. Sci. 113:* 578-594.

Forrest, G. L. and Klevecz, R. R. (1972). *J. Biol. Chem. 247:* 3147-3152.

Fouquet, H. and Braun, R. (1974). *FEBS Letters 38:* 184-186.

Friedman, D. L. (1970). *Biochem. Biophys. Res. Comm. 39:* 100-109.

Frindel, E. and Tubiana, M. (1971). In *The Cell Cycle and Cancer*, R. Baserga Ed., Marcel Dekker, New York, pp. 389-447.

Gefter, M. L., Hirota, Y., Kornberg, A., Wechsler, J. A., and Barnoux, C. (1971). *Proc. Natl. Acad. Sci. 68:* 3150-3153.

Gonzalez-Fernandez, A., Gimenez-Martin, G., Diez, J. L., De La Torre, C., and Lopez-Saez, J. F. (1971). *Chromosome 36:* 100-111.

Grisham, J. W. (1962). *Cancer Res. 22:* 842-849.

Gurdon, J. B., Birnstiel, M. L., and Speight, V. A. (1969). *Biochim. Biophys. Acta. 174:* 614-628.

Gurley, L. R. and Hardin, J. M. (1968). *Arch. Biochem. Biophys. 128:* 285-292.

Gurley, L. R. and Hardin, J. M. (1970). *Arch. Biochem. Biophys. 136:* 392-401.

Hampar, B., Tanaka, A., Nonoyama, M., and Derge, J. G. (1974). *Proc. Natl. Acad. Sci. 71:* 631-633.

Hancock, R. (1969). *J. Molec. Biol. 40:* 457-466.

Hand, R. and Tamm, I. (1974). *J. Molec. Biol. 82:* 175-183.

von Hippel, P. H. and McGhee, J. D. (1972). *Ann. Rev. Biochem. 41:* 231-300.

Hirota, Y., Mordoh, J., Scheffler, I., and Jacob, F. (1972). *Fed. Proc. 31:* 1422-1427.

Hori, T. and Lark K. G. (1973). *J. Mol. Biol. 77:* 391-404.

Huberman, J. A., Tsai, A., and Deich, R. A. (1973). *Nature 241:* 32-36.

Lambert, W. C., and Studzinski, G. P. (1969). *J. Cell. Physiol. 73:* 261-266.

Lark, K. G. (1972). *J. Mol. Biol. 64:* 47-60.

Larsson, A. (1969). *Eur. J. Biochem. 11:* 113-121.

Lesher, S., Fry, R. J. M., and Kohn, H. I. (1961). *Exp. Cell Res. 24:* 334-343.

Ley, K. D. and Tobey, R. A. (1970). *J. Cell Biol. 47:* 453-459.

Lipkin, M., Sherlock, P., and Bell, B. M. (1962). *Nature 195:* 175-177.

Malaise, E., Frindel, E., and Tubiana, M. (1967). *C. R. Acad. Sci. Paris 264:* 1104-1106.

Marks, D. B., Paik, W. K., and Borun, T. W. (1973). *J. Biol. Chem. 248:* 5660-5667.

Masker, W. E. and Eberle, H. (1971). *Proc. Natl. Acad. Sci. 68:* 2549-2553.

Moorhead, P.S. and Defendi, V. (1963). *J. Cell. Biol. 16:* 202-209.

Morishima, A., Grumbach, M. M., and Taylor, J. H. (1962). *Proc. Natl. Acad. Sci. 48:* 756-763.

Moses, R. E., Campbell, J. L., Fleishman, R. A., Frenkel, G. D., Mulcahy, H. L., Schizuya, H., and Richardson, C. C. (1972). *Fed. Proc. 31:* 1415-1421.

Mueller, G. C. (1971). In *The Cell Cycle and Cancer*, R. Baserga (Ed.). Marcel Dekker, New York, pp. 269-307.

Nias, A. H. W. and Fox, M. (1971). *Cell Tissue Kinet. 4:* 375-398.

Nicolini, C. and Baserga, R. (1974). *Exp. Molec. Pathol. 21:* 74-87.

Painter, R. B. (1961). *J. Biophys. Biochem. Cytol. 11:* 485-488.

Painter, R. B. and Rasmussen, R. E. (1964). *Nature 201:* 162-165.

Pearson, G. D. and Hanawalt, P. C. (1971). *J. Molec. Biol. 62:* 65-80.

Pedrini, A. M., Nuzzo, F., Ciarrocchi, G., Dalpra, L., and Falaschi, A. (1972). *Biochem. Biophys. Res. Comm. 47:* 1221-1227.

Prescott, D. M. (1962). *J. Histochem. Cytochem. 10:* 145-153.

Prescott, D. M. and Kuempel, P. L. (1972). *Proc. Natl. Acad. Sci. 69:* 2842-2845.

Rao, P. N and Johnson, R. T. (1970). *Nature 225:* 159-164.

Robbins, E., Jentzsch, G., and Micali, A. (1968). *J. Cell Biol. 36:* 329-339.

Sato, S., Ariake, S., Saito, M., and Sugimura, T. (1972). *Biochem. Biophys. Res. Comm. 49:* 827-834.

Sato, S., Tanaka, M., and Sugimura, T. (1970). *Biochim. Biophys. Acta. 209:* 43-48.

Sheehy, P. F., Wakonig-Vaartaja, T., Winn, R., and Clarkson, B. D. (1974). *Cancer Res. 34:* 991-996.

Spadari, S. and Weissbach, A. (1974). *J. Mol. Biol. 86:* 11-20.

Stambrook, P. J. (1974). *J. Molec. Biol. 82:* 303-313.

Stein, G. and Baserga, R. (1970). *Biochem. Biophys. Res. Comm. 41:* 715-722.

Stein, G. and Borun, T. (1972). *J. Cell Biol. 52:* 292-307.

Stryckmans, P., Cronkite, E. P., Fache, J., Fliedner, T. M., and Ramos, J. (1966). *Nature 211:* 717-720.

Stubblefield, E. (1973). *Int. Rev. Cytol. 35:* 1-60.

Stubblefield, E. and Mueller, G. C. (1962). *Cancer Res. 22:* 1091-1099.

Studzinski, G. P. and Lambert, W. C. (1969). *J. Cell. Physiol. 73:* 109-117.

Tait, R. C. and Smith, D. W. (1974). *Nature 249:* 116-119.

Taylor, J. H. (1960). *J. Biophys. Biochem. Cytol. 7:* 455-463.

Terasima, T. and Tolmach, L. J. (1963). *Exp. Cell Res. 30:* 344-362.

Tsanev, R. and Russev, G. (1974). *Eur. J. Biochem. 43:* 257-263.

Wickner, W., Brutlag, D., Schekman, R., and Kornberg, T. (1972).*Proc. Natl. Acad. Sci. 69:* 965-969.

Zampetti-Bosseler, F., Malpoix, P., and Fievez, M. (1969). *Eur. J. Biochem. 9:* 21-26.

THREE

G₂ AND MITOSIS

MACROMOLECULAR SYNTHESIS IN G₂

When DNA replication is completed, the cell progresses into the G_2 phase. During this phase, the cell synthesizes certain proteins and RNA molecules that are necessary for the continuous flow of cells from G_2 into mitosis. Tobey et al. (1971) have reviewed in detail the available information on macromolecular synthesis in G_2, and I will limit myself here to a brief summary of their discussion and to a few additional findings. After the first original report by Kishimoto and Lieberman (1964), a number of studies were carried out on the effects of inhibitors of macromolecular synthesis on G_2 cells, and the evidence indicates that inhibition of either protein or RNA synthesis during G_2 prevents the flow of cells into mitosis. The time of synthesis of the last protein(s) required for entrance into mitosis varies in different cells. It varies from 2 hours before mitosis in cells of the rat intestinal crypts to 5 minutes before mitosis in Chinese hamster cells in culture (Tobey et al. 1971). There are also indications that some of the proteins synthesized during G_2 are specific for that phase and are necessary for the orderly progression of subsequent mitosis. Jockusch et al. (1970) reported the appearance in gel electropherograms of nuclear proteins from G_2 cells of *Physarum polycephalum* a protein (or a class of proteins) not detectable in other phases of the cell cycle. Sisken and Wilkes (1967) have shown that when G_2 cells are exposed to p-fluorophenylalanine, an amino acid analog that is incorporated into proteins in place of phenylalanine, the length of mitosis is markedly prolonged. When cells are exposed to p-fluorphenylala-nine in other phases of the cell cycle, mitosis is not affected. At appropriate concentrations, p-fluorophenylalanine incorporated during the G_2 period, effectively prevents the entrance of cells into mitosis (Wheatley and Henderson 1974). The synthesis of mi-crotubular proteins, which, as mentioned in chapter 2, begins in the S phase is completed during G_2 (Forrest and Klevecz 1972). The synthesis of proteins prior to mitosis should not make us for-get that modification of preexisting proteins may be just as impor-tant. Thus, phosphorylation of nonhistone nuclear proteins reaches a minimum during late G_2 (Karn et al. 1974), while the phosphor-ylation of F_1 histone continues as in the S phase so that prior to mitosis, F_1 histone is maximally phosphorylated (Marks et al. 1973). In fact, according to Bradbury et al. (1974a and b), the phosphorylation of F_1 histone represents the initiation step for mitosis.

RNA synthesis is also required for the entry of cells into mi-tosis and, again, Tobey et al. (1971) determined, in various cell populations, the time of synthesis of the last RNA species neces-sary for the progression of cells from G_2 into mitosis. This time varies from 5 to 6 hours in Ehrlich ascites tumor cells to 30 min-utes in Chinese hamster cells. Attempts to further identify these putative messenger RNA species associated with the entry of cells into mitosis have thus far not been successful.

INHIBITORS OF G_2

Besides the above-mentioned inhibitors of macromole-cular synthesis, other substances have been reported that are capa-ble of arresting cells in G_2. A good example of such a substance (with tissue specificity) is isoproterenol, which has been shown by Radley and Hodgson (1971) to block temporarily, in G_2 or meta-phase, acinar cells of the parotid. Since isoproterenol is a powerful β -adrenergic agent capable of stimulating adenyl cyclase and of increasing intracellular levels of cyclic AMP (Durham et al. 1974), one would predict that cyclic AMP could cause arrest of cells in G_2. Indeed, cyclic AMP has been reported to cause G_2 arrest both in human lymphoid cells (Millis et al. 1972) and in Chinese hamster ovary cells (Remington and Klevecz 1973). In addition, intracellular cyclic AMP levels are increased during G_2 (Millis et al. 1972). Chalones have also been implicated as inhibitors of the flow of cells from G_2 to mitosis. For instance, chalones capable of producing the arrest of G_2 have been reported in the epidermis (Bullough and Laurence 1964), in the kidney, and in lymphocytes (see review by Houck and Hennings 1973). Similarly, an epidermal chalone, isolated by Argyris (1972) from mammalian skin and exhibiting partial tissue specificity, prevented G_2 cells from entering mitosis. Although this chalone had the properties of a glycoprotein, in general, the nature of the regulatory molecules of the G_2 phase (whether RNA, proteins, isoproterenol, or chalones) is largely obscure.

Probably related to chalones is the finding, in fusion experiments, that the presence of S nuclei delays the entrance of G_2 nuclei into mitosis (Rao and Johnson 1970). Finally, it should be mentioned that certain hormones, such as the melanocyte stimulating hormone, are capable of binding to target cells only in the G_2 phase (Varga et al. 1974).

LENGTH OF G_2 AND MITOSIS

The length of G_2 and mitosis in some mammalian cells, in vivo and in vitro, is given in Table 3.1. The difference in the length of G_2 between normal and cancerous cells will be discussed further in chapter 13.

MEMBRANE CHANGES IN MITOSIS

A bit more information is available on the biochemical basis of mitosis itself, in its four stages from prophase to telophase. The striking cytological changes associated with the formation of

TABLE 3.1   Duration of G_2 and Mitosis in Representative Mammalian Cells

Cell type	Duration (hr) of G_2	Mitosis	Reference
Crypt epithelium of mouse small intestine		1.38	Fry et al. (1961)
Crypt epithelium of rat small intestine		0.43	Wright et al. (1972)
Mouse embryo primitive ependymal cells	1.0	1.00	Atlas and Bond (1965)
Regenerating rat liver	2.5		Fabrikant (1968)
Morris hepatoma 5123 tc	3-15		Sasaki et al. (1970)
Epithelial cells, man, colon	1.0		Lipkin et al. (1962)
Metastatic carcinoma of ovary, man	3-16		Clarkson et al. (1965)
HeLa S_3 cells	3.0		Terasima and Tolmach (1963)
L-mouse cells	4.8		Cleaver (1965)
Human diploid fibroblasts	4.0		Defendi and Manson (1963)
Cultured human lymphocytes	3.5		Cave (1966)

the mitotic apparatus have, of course, been known for nearly 100 years, but recently some information has also been obtained concerning its chemical nature. It now seems apparent that the proteins involved in the formation of the mitotic spindle are proteins from the microtubules (synthesized during the latter part of S and G_2) and that the function of these contractile proteins may largely depend on the number of SH groups. Since the energy requirements for mitosis have also been discussed in detail by Tobey et al. (1971), I will discuss here briefly only the events occurring on the cell membrane and the changes in macromolecular synthesis that occur during mitosis itself.

Changes in the surface membranes of mitotic cells have been described for more than 25 years, Heilbrunn (1956) being the first to propose that changes in the cell cortex may be attributed to a loss of Ca^{++} ions from the cell surface. Subsequently, it was shown that the electrophoretic mobility of cells in culture increased sharply when cells entered mitosis and dropped precipitously at the completion of telophase (Mayhew 1966). The net negative charge of the cell surface is partially due to the charged COOH groups of sialic acid and, in fact, removal of sialic acid by neuraminidase eliminates the rise in electrophoretic mobility at mitosis. Kraemer (1967), however, believes that the elevation in electrophoretic mobility at mitosis is due to conformational changes of sialoglycolipids or sialoglycopeptides on the cell surface rather than to a change in surface density of terminal sialic acid molecules. Subsequently, Kraemer and Tobey (1972) reported, in Chinese hamster ovary cells, that just prior to mitosis there is a loss of surface heparin sulfate, a mucopolysaccharide with a structure similar to heparin but which lacks significant anticoagulant potency.

Also of considerable interest have been the findings of Burger and coworkers (Burger and Goldberg 1967, Fox et al. 1971), on the ability of certain plant agglutinins to bind to the cell surface of interphase and mitotic cells. Thus, both wheat germ agglutinin and concanavalin A do not agglutinate normal cells in culture, although they bind to and agglutinate virus-transformed cells or tumor cells (this will be discussed in more detail in chapter 9). However, when normal cells are in mitosis they can be agglutinated by plant agglutinins, like transformed cells cells. Related to this phenomenon is the finding of Glick and Buck (1973) that glycopeptides expressed on the cell surface during mitosis are similar to those permanently expressed after viral transformation. The report that cells in mitosis have a greater ability to undergo Sendai virus-induced fusion than do cells in interphase further supports the concept of structural and functional changes in the membranes of mitotic cells (Stadler and Adelberg 1972). Indeed, diploid chicken embryo cells, which are capable of proliferation only as monolayers on artificial surfaces, become arrested in G_2 (Yaoi et al. 1972) when placed in suspension cultures (which causes changes in membrane structure). Separate from, but somewhat related to membranes, are microfilaments. Their importance has been highlighted by the mold metabolite cytochalasin B, which, by dissociating microfilaments in the cleavage furrow, inhibits cytokinesis (Wright and Hayflick 1972, Kelly and Sambrook 1973).

PROTEIN SYNTHESIS DURING MITOSIS

During mitosis the rate of protein synthesis is markedly decreased (Baserga 1962, Scharff and Robbins 1966, Prescott 1962). However, different classes of proteins are affected differently. For instance, while histone synthesis completely ceases and the rate of synthesis of total cellular proteins is about 20% of the rate observed in interphase cells, the rate of synthesis of nonhistone chromosomal proteins continues during mitosis at the same rate as in interphase (Stein and Baserga 1970). There are contradictory views on the mechanism responsible for the marked decrease in the rate of protein synthesis during mitosis in mammalian cells. Salb and Marcus (1965) believed that the decreased synthetic capacity was due to a modification of the polyribosomes, more specifically to a coating of ribosomes with a trypsin-sensitive material possibly derived from the nucleus. Johnson and Holland (1965), however, found that the ribosomes of mitotic cells supported protein synthesis as efficiently as interphase ribosomes, if a synthetic messenger RNA, for instance poly U, was added. This observation, coupled with the fact that normal yields of poliovirus were produced in metaphase-arrested cells, led Johnson and Holland (1965) to conclude that the reduced rate of protein synthesis during mitosis was due to the unavailability of messenger RNA to ribosomes. The fact that the synthesis of only certain types of proteins is inhibited during mitosis seems to support Johnson and Holland's theory that unavailability of messenger RNA rather than

aspecific changes in ribosomes may be responsible for the decrease
in the rate of protein synthesis. These two views could be reconciled by the findings of Fan and Penman (1970) that in Chinese
hamster ovary cells in mitosis ribosomes become attached to messenger RNA and initiate polypeptide synthesis at a reduced rate.

                     RNA SYNTHESIS DURING MITOSIS

        The rate of RNA synthesis is also decreased during mito-
sis, and, in fact, as observed several years ago by Taylor (1960),
RNA synthesis ceases during metaphase and anaphase. Taylor's observation has been confirmed by a number of investigators (see review by Prescott 1964), and it constitutes one of the most fascin-
ating models for the study of gene expression. During mitosis,
DNA transcription comes to a standstill, and it would certainly be
relevant to our understanding of gene expression to identify the
factors that inhibit DNA transcription during mitosis. This model
has not received all the attention that it deserves, probably because a considerable number of investigators have felt that changes
in DNA transcription during mitosis may not be typical of gene
regulation in mammalian cells. Even so, the model still remains ex-
remely attractive, especially in light of the findings of Johnson and
Holland (1965). These authors found that while DNA extracted
from mitotic or interphase cells served equally well as template for
an exogenous *E. coli* RNA polymerase, deoxyribonucleoprotein
from mitotic cells was a much less efficient template for purified
E. coli RNA polymerase than is deoxyribonucleoprotein from interphase cells. These studies suggested that the decrease in RNA
synthesis in mitotic cells was due to the proteins of the chromosome. Johnson and Holland's (1965) results have been confirmed
by Farber et al. (1972) who showed that the template activity of
chromatin from mitotic cells is only about 20% of that of chromatin from S-phase cells. In addition, when DNA extracted from log-
phase cells was reconstituted with chromosomal proteins from
either S-phase cells or mitotic cells, the template activity of the reconstituted chromatin was higher when S-phase proteins were used

for the reconstitution than when proteins from mitotic cells were used (the validity of chromatin reconstitution experiments will be discussed in a later chapter). These results indicate that the supression of RNA synthesis during mitosis is due to proteins of the chromatin. Whether these proteins cause a conformational change in the DNA molecule is not known. The important point is that chromosomal proteins are the determinants of template activity in mitotic cells, and it is to be hoped that in the future this model will be more extensively used to investigate the mechanisms of gene expression. The potential of this model has already been confirmed by the report, also using reconstituted chromatins, that the chromosomal proteins responsible for the decreased template activity of mitotic chromatin may be nonhistone chromosomal proteins (Stein and Farber 1972). However, a possible alternative could be offered by the finding of Lake and Salzman (1972) that in mitotic cells there is a marked increase (in respect to interphase cells) of a chromatin-associated phosphokinase having high specificity for F_1 histone.

We will not discuss here the structure of chromosomes, a topic that goes beyond the range of this monograph. For the interested reader we would like to recommend two excellent reviews that have appeared recently, one by Huberman (1973) and the other by Stubblefield (1973).

DNA SYNTHESIS AND MITOSIS

The next question we would like to ask is "What is the relationship of DNA synthesis to cell division"? In other words, is cell division strictly dependent on previous DNA synthesis or can the two processes be separated and occur independently? In bacteria it is stated that cell division is controlled by DNA replication and that termination of DNA replication triggers a cycle of division (Lark 1969). The contrary is not true; that is, at least in bacteria, cell division does not appear to regulate replication of DNA. A similar situation occurs in yeasts, where Hartwell (1971) studied the behavior of two temperature-sensitive mutants of *Saccharo-*

myces cerevisiae. One of the mutants was defective in the initiation of DNA replication and the other in the continuation of DNA replication at the restrictive temperature. On the basis of his investigations with these mutants, Hartwell (1971) concluded that in yeast nuclear division and cell separation depend on prior DNA replication. In mammalian cells, however, there is no formal demonstration that the cessation of DNA synthesis actually triggers mitosis. We may say, however, that the two processes are usually correlated and that in the great majority of cases mitosis is preceded by DNA synthesis and, conversely, completion of DNA replication leads to mitosis. After stating this rule, the least we can do is find out the inevitable exceptions of which there are, in fact, a great number. Some lower animals, like the small freshwater coelenterate *Hydra attenuata*, think that G_2 is the only place to stay. Thus Hydra epithelial cells have a G_2 period that lasts 48 to 72 hours, while $S + G_1$ + mitosis amount to a mere 14 hours (David and Campbell 1972). But the obvious exception in which we are interested is the existence of tetraploid cells, that is, cells with an amount of DNA double that of the diploid amount proper for the species. Tetraploid cells are obviously cells that have replicated their DNA without dividing. However, the credit must go to Gelfant (1963) for pointing out that at least in certain tissues there are a number of cells that have been arrested in the G_2 phase of the cell cycle from which they can be stimulated to enter directly mitosis if an appropriate stimulus is given. This is a different situation from tetraploid cells. For instance, there is a large fraction of tetraploid cells in the liver, yet, when the liver regenerates after partial hepatectomy tetraploid cells enter DNA synthesis before they divide again into two daughter tetraploid cells. In the case of G_2-arrested cells, one is dealing with cells that, although tetraploid, will proceed directly to mitosis, if a proliferating stimulus is applied.

We will discuss the concept of tetraploidy and hypertrophy in chapter 12. For the moment we shall limit ourselves to observe that in mammalian cells DNA synthesis and mitosis can occasionally be independent from each other, although in the great majority of cases a DNA-synthesizing cell is a cell already committed to divide.

REFERENCES

Argyris, T. S. (1972). *Am. Zoologist 12:* 137-149.
Atlas, M. and Bond, V. P. (1965). *J. Cell Biol. 26:* 19-24.
Baserga, R. (1962). *Biochim. Biophys. Acta. 61:* 445-450.
Bradbury, E. M., Inglis, R. J., and Matthews, H. R. (1974a). *Nature 247:* 257-261.
Bradbury, E. M., Inglis, R. J., Matthews, H. R., and Langan, T. A. (1974b). *Nature 249:* 553-556.
Bullough, W. S. and Laurence, E. B. (1964). *Exp. Cell Res. 33:* 176-194.
Burger, M. M. and Goldberg, A. R..(1967). *Proc. Natl. Acad. Sci. USA 57:* 359-366.
Cave, MacD. (1966). *J. Cell Biol. 29:* 209-222.
Clarkson, B., Ota, K., Ohkita, T., and O'Connor, A. (1965). *Cancer 18:* 1189-1213.
Cleaver, J. E. (1965). *Exp. Cell Res. 39:* 697-700.
David, C. N. and Campbell, R. D. (1972). *J. Cell Sci. 11:* 557-568.
Defendi, V. and Manson, L. A. (1963). *Nature 198:* 359-361.
Durham, J. P., Baserga, R., and Butcher, F. R. (1974). In *Control of Proliferation in Animal Cells*, B. Clarkson and R. Baserga (Eds.). Cold Spring Harbor Laboratory, pp. 595-607.
Fabrikant, J. I. (1968). *J. Cell Biol. 36:* 551-565.
Fan, H. and Penman, S. (1970). *J. Mol. Biol. 50:* 655-670.
Farber, J., Stein, G., and Baserga, R. (1972). *Biochem. Biophys. Res. Comm. 47:* 790-797.
Forrest, G. L. and Klevecz, R. R. (1972). *J. Biol. Chem. 247:* 3147-3152.
Fox, T. O., Sheppard, J. R., and Burger, M. M. (1971). *Proc. Natl. Acad. Sci. USA 68:* 244-247.
Fry, R. J. N., Lesher, S., and Kohn, H. I. (1961). *Nature 191:* 290-291.
Gelfant, S. (1963). *Int. Rev. Cytolol. 14:* 1-39.
Glick, M. C. and Buck, C. A. (1973). *Biochemistry 12:* 85-90.
Hartwell, L. H. (1971). *J. Mol. Biol. 59:* 183-194.
Heilbrunn, L. V. (1956). *The Dynamics of Living Protoplasm.* Academic Press, New York.
Houck, J. C. and Hennings, H. (1973). *FEBS Letters 32:* 1-8.
Huberman, J. A. (1973). *Ann. Rev. Biochem. 42:* 355-378.

Jockusch, B. M., Brown, D. F., and Rusch, H. P. (1970). *Biochem. Biophys. Res. Comm. 38:* 279-283.

Johnson, D. C. and Holland, J. J. (1965). *J. Cell Biol. 27:* 565-574.

Karn, J., Johnson, E. M., Vidali, G., and Allfrey, V. G. (1974). *J. Biol. Chem. 249:* 667-677.

Kelly, F. and Sambrook, J. (1973). *Nature New Biol. 242:* 217-219.

Kishimoto, S. and Lieberman, I. (1964). *Exp. Cell Res. 36:* 92-101.

Kraemer, P. M. (1967). *J. Cell Biol. 33:* 197-200.

Kraemer, P. M. and Tobey, R. A. (1972). *J. Cell Biol. 55:* 713-717.

Lake, R. S. and Salzman, N. P. (1972). *Biochemistry 11:* 4817-4826.

Lark, K. G. (1969). *Ann Rev. Biochem. 38:* 569-604.

Lipkin, M., Sherlock, P., and Bell, B. M. (1962). *Nature 195:* 175-177.

Marks, D., Paik, W. K., and Borun, T. W. (1973). *J. Biol. Chem. 248:* 5660-5667.

Mayhew, E. (1966). *J. Gen. Physiol. 49:* 717-725.

Millis, A. J. T., Forrest, G., and Pious, D. A. (1972). *Biochem. Biophys. Res. Comm. 49:* 1645-1649.

Prescott, D. M. (1962). *J. Histochem. Cytochem. 10:* 145-153.

Prescott, D. M. (1964). Cellular sites of RNA synthesis. In *Progress of nucleic Acid Research and Molecular Biology*, J. N. Davidson and W. E. Cohn (Eds.). Academic Press, New York, p. 33.

Radley, J. M. and Hodgson, G. S. (1971). *Exp. Cell Res. 69:* 148-160.

Rao, P. N. and Johnson, R. T. (1970). *Nature 225:* 159-164.

Remington, J. A. and Klevecz, R. R. (1973). *Biochem. Biophys. Res. Comm. 50:* 140-146.

Salb, J. M. and Marcus, P. I. (1965). *Proc. Natl. Acad. Sci. USA 54:* 1353-1358.

Sasaki, T., Morris, H. P., and Baserga, R. (1970). *Cancer Res. 30:* 788-793.

Scharff, M. D. and Robbins, E. (1966). *Science 151:* 992-995.

Sisken, J. E. and Wilkes, E. (1967). *J. Cell Biol. 34:*97-110.

Stadler, J. K. and Adelberg, E. A. (1972). *Proc. Natl. Acad. Sci. USA 69:* 1929-1933.

Stein, G. and Baserga, R. (1970). *Biochem. Biophys. Res. Comm. 41:* 715-722.

Stein, G. and Farber, J. (1972). *Proc. Natl. Acad. Sci. USA 69:* 2918-2921.

Stubblefield, E. (1973). *Int. Rev. Cytol. 35:* 1-60.

Taylor, J. H. (1960). *Ann. N. Y. Acad. Sci. 90:* 409-421.

Terasima, T. and Tolmach, L. J. (1963). *Exp. Cell Res. 30:* 344-362.

Tobey, R. A., Petersen, D. F., and Anderson, E. C. (1971). Biochemistry of G_2 and mitosis. In *The Cell Cycle and Cancer*, R. Baserga (Ed.). Marcel Dekker, New York, pp. 309-353.

Varga, J. M., DiPasquale, A., Pawelek, J., McGuire, J. S., and Lerner, A. B. (1974). *Proc. Natl. Acad. Sci. USA 71:* 1590-1593.
Wheatley, D. N. and Henderson, J. Y. (1974). *Nature 247:* 281-283.
Wright, W. E. and Hayflick, L. (1972). *Exp. Cell Res. 74:* 187-194.
Wright, N., Morley, A., and Appleton, D. (1972). *Cell Tissue Kinet. 5:* 351-364.
Yaoi, Y., Onoda, T., and Takahashi, H. (1972). *Nature 237:* 285-286.

FOUR

G$_1$ PHASE

RNA SYNTHESIS

Investigations on the biochemistry of G$_1$ cells have also been facilitated by the use of synchronized cells in culture, and in recent years some fragmentary knowledge has begun to emerge on biochemical events occurring in G$_1$ cells that are related to the subsequent onset of DNA synthesis. Actually, the oldest and still significant bit of information on the biochemistry of G$_1$ was obtained with an asynchronous population of cells. This study was based on a previous observation by Lieberman et al. (1963) whose importance will be discussed in a later chapter on explanted rabbit kidney cells. These quiescent cells enter DNA synthesis after a lag period of about 30 hours or more after explantation. Lieberman and coworkers (1963) found that the entrance of rabbit kidney cells into DNA synthesis was inhibited when the explants were exposed to small amounts of actinomycin D (0.1 μg/ml or less). Baserga and coworkers (1965a and b) applied these findings to continuously-dividing cells and investigated the effect of small doses of actinomycin D (0.016 μg/g of body weight) on the cell cycle of Ehrlich ascites tumor cells growing asynchronously in the peritoneal cavity of mice. They found that this small dose of actinomycin D did not inhibit DNA synthesis per se nor the flow of cells

44

through G_2. However, the regular flow of cells from G_1 into S was inhibited. In fact, by analyzing the kinetics of the inhibitory effect, Baserga and coworkers were able to locate this actinomycin-D-sensitive step (which could reasonably be considered as a step requiring RNA synthesis) at a G_1 point situated 3 hours before the onset of DNA synthesis. The original findings of Baserga and coworkers have been subsequently confirmed by a number of investigators in a great variety of tissues, both in vitro (see review by Doida and Okada 1972) and in vivo, (Baserga et al. 1966) indicating that the synthesis of some kind of RNA species is a prerequisite for the progression of cells from G_1 to S. Perhaps related to the requirement for RNA synthesis is the report of Pederson (1972) that chromatin isolated from HeLa cells in late G_1 binds more actinomycin D and is less resistant to digestion with DNase I than chromatin from other phases of the cell cycle.

PROTEIN SYNTHESIS

A requirement for protein synthesis was demonstrated in 1966 by Terasima and Yasukawa using synchronized mouse-L cells. G_1 cells were obtained by mitotic selection and the time required to enter DNA synthesis (after mitotic selection) was determined. Terasima and Yasukawa (1966) showed that the interval between completion of mitosis and onset of DNA synthesis was delayed by 2 hours if G_1 cells (anywhere in the G_1 period) were exposed for 2 hours to an inhibitor of protein synthesis. Their results indicated that an undisturbed synthesis of proteins throughout the G_1 period is necessary for the entrance of cells into S. The effect of inhibitors of macromolecular synthesis on the progression of cells from G_1 to S has been reviewed and studied in detail by Doida and Okada (1972). They conclude that ". . . two conditions have to be fulfilled for the cells' entry into S stage: one is synthesis of new messenger RNA at the beginning of the G_1 stage and the second is synthesis of new proteins (sometimes called G_1 proteins)." In essence, most investigators will accept these two requirements for RNA and protein synthesis as the critical steps for the progression of cells from G_1 to S. However, neither event has been elucidated in much greater detail than in the two original experiments, and both the necessary RNA species and the necessary protein species have yet to be isolated and identified. Thus, although some of the steps occurring in G_1 are recognizable, the information is only vague. Perhaps the use of temperature-sensitive mutants will increase our chances to identify these unknown macromolecules (see below).

OTHER BIOCHEMICAL EVENTS

Some other events occurring in G_1 have been described and are listed in Table 4.1. However, the relationship of these events to the subsequent onset of DNA synthesis is reasonably established only for the first five events listed. Histone phosphorylation and, more specifically, phosphorylation of F_1 histone, although beginning in mammalian cells at the end of the G_1 period, is probably more related to mitosis than to the onset of DNA synthesis (see chapter 3).

Despite the fact that the G_1-restricted cytotoxicity of antibodies to Moloney virus-transformed lymphocytes is probably not specifically related to the control of DNA synthesis, it is of considerable interest because it points out that cells may have different sensitivities in different phases of the cell cycle. In this particular case viral antigen was present on the cell surface; it was accessible to antibody and able to activate complement in the presence of antibody throughout all cellular growth phases and yet immunolysis occurred only during G_1. The importance of this observation in terms of immunotherapy can hardly be overemphasized. Yet, one should remember that although large doses are cytotoxic, brief exposure to small doses of antibodies specific for cell surface antigens stimulates the growth of cells in suspension (Shearer et al. 1973). Of particular interest are the changes in membrane function occurring in G_1 cells. Both Sander and Pardee (1972) and Costlow et al. (1973) have shown that the uptake of low molecular weight compounds (such as amino acids and nucleo-

TABLE 4.1   Biochemistry of G_1 Period

Molecular Event	References
Synthesis of specific RNA	Baserga et al. (1965a), Doida and Okada (1972)
Synthesis of specific proteins	Terasima and Yasukawa (1966), Doida and Okada (1972)
Synthesis of histone mRNA	Borun et al. (1967)
Lack of thymidine kinase	Brent et al. (1965), Stubblefield and Mueller (1965)
Lack of dCMP deaminase	Gelbard et al (1969)
Noninducibility of TAT	Martin et al. (1969)
Synthesis of immunoglobulins	Buell and Fahey (1969)
Reformation of polyribosomes	Steward et al. (1968)
K^+ and Na^+ changes	Jung and Rothstein (1967)
Cytotoxicity of antibodies	Lerner et al. (1971)
Phosphorylation of histones	Balhorn et al. (1972), Marks et al. (1973)
Sensitivity to oncogenic transformation	Bertram and Heidelberger (1974)
Increased pool of deoxynucleotides	Tobey et al. (1974)

sides) increases after mitosis. When the cells are arrested in G_1, as for instance, by starvation, release of the block causes an immediate increase in the uptake of low molecular weight compounds. These changes will be discussed in more detail in later chapters, when the role of membranes in cell proliferation (chapter 9) will be considered and G_1 cells will be compared to G_0 cells (chapter 11). Also to be mentioned briefly are the reports of G_1-specific chalones, ie., of cellular substances that inhibit the flow of cells from G_1 to S. Chalones inhibitory for G_1 cells have been described in epidermis, liver, melanocytes, and fibroblasts (see review by Houck and Hennings 1973).

An interesting feature of the G_1 cells is that they are more sensitive to oncogenic transformation by the mutagen N-Methyl-N'-nitro-N-nitrosoguanidine (Bertram and Heidelberger 1974). The interest lies in the fact that several temperature-sensitive mutants have been recently described that are cell cycle specific (see also chapter 6), that is, they stop growing at the non-permissive temperature at a specific point in the cell cycle. In several of these cell-cycle temperature-sensitive mutants the sensitive step is in late G_1 (Burstin et al. 1975, Roscoe et al. 1973, Liskay 1974). Whether this is due to the fact that N-methyl-N'-nitro-N-nitrosoguanidine was also used to obtain the mutants, or that late G_1 has a step exquisitely sensitive to mutation and onco-genic transformation remains to be determined.

Tobey et al. (1974), besides confirming the increased phosphorylation of F_1 histone, have reported, in the late G_1 of CHO cells, an increase in membrane-DNA complex formation and an increase in deoxynucleotide triphosphate pools.

The problem of size must still be discussed. The hypothesis that cell division is triggered by a critical cell mass recurs in biology with the regularity of a malarial fever. While some of the

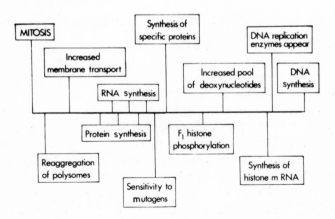

FIGURE 4.1   Diagram of cell cycle-specific events in the G_1 period of mammalian cells.

evidence marshalled to support this hypothesis is certainly based on sound observations, most of the data indicate that cells grow in size because they are going to divide, and not vice versa. The growth of cells in preparation for cell division will be analyzed in detail in the chapter on G_0 cells. Suffice it to say here that the demonstration by Fox and Pardee (1970) that the heterogeneity in the length of G_1 in mammalian cells is not due to variations in cell size, indicates that a critical mass is not needed for the regular flow of cells in the cell cycle. Or, to borrow the wisdom of an old Pennsylvania Dutch proverb: "It does not depend on size, or a cow could catch a rabbit."

CONCLUSIONS

In summary, while the synchronization of cells in culture in G_1 is feasible and some events occurring in the G_1 period have been identified, we know very little about the specific macromolecules synthesized in the G_1 phase that control the flow of cells from G_1 to S. In fact, the available data seem to indicate that the RNA species necessary for the flow of cells from G_1 to S may be ribosomal RNA. This is based on the often-repeated observation (mentioned above) that there is a step in G_1 sensitive to very low doses of actinomycin D, which are supposed to inhibit specifically the synthesis of ribosomal RNA (Perry and Kelley 1968). Also, at variance with G_0 cells stimulated to synthesize DNA and divide, no evidence has yet been brought forward that gene activation is required. Thus, no changes in chromatin template activity have been observed in cells arrested in G_1 and subsequently stimulated to proliferate, as for instance 3T6 mouse fibroblasts (Rovera and Baserga 1973), and SV-40 transformed WI-38 human diploid fibroblasts (Costlow and Baserga 1973). It should be noted, at this point, that the reaggregation of polysomes and restoration of protein synthesis that occur when mitotic cells enter G_1 are both under translational control. The step takes place even in the presence of high doses of actinomycin D and apprently does not require the synthesis of any new messenger RNA (Steward et al.

1968, Hodge et al. 1969). In fact, after mitosis, the return of the rate of RNA synthesis to interphase levels is even independent of protein synthesis, although its maintenance during G_1 requires renewed protein synthesis (Simmons et al. 1973, see also review by Doida and Okada, 1972). If this were true, then the difference between G_1 and G_0 cells may be based on a fundamental difference, ie., the activation of new gene sites. These differences and the possible controlling mechanisms will be discussed again when we compare G_1 to G_0 in chapter 11. As a preview of such a comparison, Table 4.2 gives the length of G_1 and G_0 phases in some representative mammalian cells; Fig. 4.1 gives a schematic diagram of the relevant biochemical events occurring in the G_1 period.

TABLE 4.2   Duration of G_1 (or G_0) in Representative Mammalian Cells

G_1	Hours[a]	Reference
Mouse embryo primitive ependymal cells	3.5	Atlas and Bond (1965)
L mouse cells	6.2	Cleaver (1965)
Sheep, wool follicles	9	Downes et al. (1966)
Mammary gland of mouse, alveoli	38	Bresciani (1968)
Mouse ascites tumor	2.5-15	Frindel et al. (1968)
Human diploid fibroblasts	6	Macieira-Coelho et al. (1966)
HeLa S_3	8	Terasima and Tolmach (1963)
Rat, polychromatic erythroblasts	1.0	Hanna et al. (1969)
G_0		
Human diploid fibroblasts	12-15	Farber et al. (1971)
Primary cultures of rabbit kidney cells	30-50	Lieberman et al. (1963)
Regenerating rat liver	18	Grisham (1962)
Mouse uterine epithelium castrated	31.5	Epifanova (1966)
estrone-treated	18.5	

[a] Duration of G_1 and G_0.

REFERENCES

Atlas, M. and Bond, V. P. (1965). *J. Cell Biol. 26:* 19-24.

Balhorn, R., Bordwell, J., Sellers, L., Granner, D., and Chalkley, R. (1972). *Biochem. Biophys. Res. Comm. 46:* 1326-1333.

Baserga, R., Estensen, R. D., Petersen, R. O., and Layde, J. P. (1965a). *Proc. Natl. Acad. Sci. USA 54:* 745-751.

Baserga, R., Estensen, R. D., and Petersen, R. O. (1965b). *Proc. Natl. Acad. Sci. USA 54:* 1141-1148.

Baserga, R., Estensen, R. D., and Petersen, R. O. (1966). *J. Cell Physiol. 68:* 177-184.

Bertram, J. S. and Heidelberger, C. (1974). *Cancer Res. 34:* 526-537.

Borun, T. W., Scharff, M. D., and Robbins, E. (1967). *Proc. Natl. Acad. Sci. USA 58:* 1977-1983.

Brent, T. P., Butler, J. A. V., and Crathorn, A. R. (1965). *Nature 207:* 176-177.

Bresciani, F. (1968). *Eur. J. Cancer 4:* 343-366.

Buell, D. and Fahey, J. L. (1969). *Science 164:* 1524-1525.

Burstin, S. J., Meiss, H. K., and Basilico, C. (1974). *J. Cell. Physiol. 84*:397-407.

Cleaver, J. E. (1965). *Exp. Cell Res. 39:* 697-700.

Costlow, M. and Baserga, R. (1973). *J. Cell Physiol. 82:* 411-420.

Doida, Y. and Okada, S. (1972). *Cell Tissue Kinet. 5:* 15-26.

Downes, A. M., Chapman, R. E., Till, A. R., and Wilson, P. A. (1966). *Nature 212:* 477-479.

Epifanova, O. I. (1966). *Exp. Cell Res. 42:* 562-577.

Farber, J., Rovera, G., and Baserga, R. (1971). *Biochem. J. 122:* 189-195.

Fox, T. O. and Pardee, A. B. (1970). *Science 167:* 80-82.

Frindel, E., Vassort, F., Malaise, E., Croizat, H., and Tubiana, M. (1968). *Bull. Cancer 55:* 9-20.

Gelbard, A. S., Kim, J. H., and Perez, A. G. (1969). *Biochim. Biophys. Acta 182:* 564-566.

Grisham, J. W. (1962). *Cancer Res. 22:* 842-849.

Hanna, I. R. A., Tarbutt, R. G., and Lamerton, L. F. (1969). *Br. J. Haematol. 16:* 381-387.

Hodge, L. D., Borun, T. W., Robbins, E., and Scharff, M. D. (1969). In *Biochemistry of Cell Division*, R. Baserga (Ed.). C. C. Thomas, Springfield, pp. 15-37.

Houck, J. C. and Hennings, H. (1973). *FEBS Letters 32:* 1-8.

Jung, C. and Rothstein, A. (1967). *J. Gen. Physiol. 50:* 917-932.

Lerner, R. A., Goldstone, M. B. A., and Cooper, N. R. (1971). *Proc. Natl. Acad. Sci. USA 68:* 2584-2588.

Lieberman, I., Abrams, R., and Ove, P. (1963). *J. Biol. Chem. 238:* 2141-2149.

Liskay, R. M. (1974). *J. Cell Physiol. 84:* 49-56

Macieira-Coelho, A., Ponten, J., and Philipson, L. (1966). *Exp. Cell Res. 42:* 673-684.

Marks, D. B., Paik, W. K., and Borun, T. W. (1973). *J. Biol. Chem. 248:* 5660-5667.

Martin, D., Jr., Tomkins, G. M., and Granner, D. (1969). *Proc. Natl. Acad. Sci. USA 62:* 248-255.

Pedersen, T. (1972). *Proc. Natl. Acad. Sci. 69:* 2224-2228.

Perry, R. P. and Kelley, D. E. (1968). *J. Cell Physiol. 72:* 235-246.

Roscoe, D. H., Robinson, H., and Carbonell, A. W. (1973). *J. Cell Physiol. 82:* 333-338.

Rovera, G. and Baserga, R. (1973). *Exp. Cell Res. 78:* 118-126.

Sander, G. and Pardee, A. B. (1972). *J. Cell Physiol. 80:* 267-272.

Shearer, W. T., Philpott, G. W., and Parker, C. W. (1973). *Science 182:* 1357-1359.

Simmons, T., Heywood, P., and Hodge, L. (1973). *J. Cell Biol. 59:* 150-164.

Steward, D. L., Shaeffer, J. R., and Humphrey, R. M. (1968). *Science 161:* 791-793.

Stubblefield, E. and Mueller, G. C. (1965). *Biochem. Biophys. Res. Comm. 20:* 535-538.

Terasima, T. and Tolmach, L. J. (1963). *Exp. Cell Res. 30:* 344-362.

Terasima, T. and Yasukawa, M. (1966). *Exp. Cell Res. 44:* 669-672.

Tobey, R. A., Gurley, L. R., Hildebrand, C. E., Ratliff, R. L., and Walters, R. A. (1974). In *Control of Proliferation in Animal Cells*, B. Clarkson and R. Baserga (Eds.). Cold Spring Harbor, pp. 665-679.

FIVE

THE PREREPLICATIVE PHASE OF G_0 CELLS

G_0 CELLS AND BACTERIAL SPORES

While continuously-dividing cells keep riding the merry-go-round of the cell cycle, other, perhaps wiser cells remain in a quiescent state from which they can be stimulated to synthesize DNA and divide by the application of an appropriate stimulus. Quiescent cells still capable of synthesizing DNA and dividing are called G_0 cells and we shall give, in chapter 11, the evidence upon which many investigators believe that G_0 cells can be distinguished from G_1 cells. For the moment, let us say that not only are there several populations of G_0 cells in the adult animal, but that the G_0 state can be reproduced in cultures, particularly in monolayer cultures (Baserga 1968). Populations of G_0 cells that can be stimulated to proliferate by an appropriate stimulus are listed in Tables 5.1 (in vitro) and 5.2 (in vivo). They have in common the following characteristics: (a) in unstimulated G_0 cells, DNA synthesis and cell division have all but ceased; (b) when quiescent cells are stimulated to proliferate, they can again synthesize DNA and divide; (c) between the application of the stimulus and the onset of DNA synthesis there is a lag period (the prereplicative phase) which varies between 6 (Temin 1971) and more than 30 hours (Taylor et al. 1966); and (d) DNA replication is an obligatory step before cell division in G_0 cells. Cells that proceed from G_2 to

mitosis should not be considered G_0 cells, and as such, they have
been discussed in chapters 1 and 3.

Anyone of the quiescent cell populations listed in Tables
5.1 and 5.2 can be utilized to increase our understanding of the
molecular basis of cell proliferation in mammalian cells. Incidentally the prereplicative phase of stimulated G_0 cells has a prokary-
otic analog in the germination of bacterial spores. Spores are dormant bacterial cells in which the genome can be brought back to
an active state by the application of an appropriate stimulus. The
sequence of biochemical events that occurs when bacterial spores
are caused to germinate has been described in detail (Kobayashi et
al. 1965) and bears a considerable resemblance to the biochemical
events that occur in the prereplicative phase of G_0 cells stimulated
to proliferate. Thus, in *Bacillus subtilis* the first detectable event in
germinating spores is the synthesis of transfer RNA and ribosomal
RNA, which begins within 2 minutes after exposure to the germinating medium. Messenger RNA and protein synthesis begin at
about 15 minutes, while DNA synthesis does not begin until 45
minutes after exposure to the germinating medium (Armstrong
and Sueoka 1968). In this system too, therefore, a lag period is
present between the application of the stimulus and the onset of
DNA synthesis, a lag period during which a number of events take
place that are of primary importance for the subsequent replication of DNA and cell division.

The mammalian cell being somewhat more complicated
than the bacterial cell, the sequence of biochemical events in the
prereplicative phase of stimulated G_0 cells is correspondingly more
elaborate. Despite its complexity and the fact that several points
are still unresolved, sufficient information is available to allow us a
reasonably adequate description of the biochemical events occurring between the application of a proliferative stimulus and mitosis. The question, then, that we shall ask ourselves in this and subsequent chapters is: "what happens in molecular terms in resting
cells stimulated to proliferate between the application of the stimulus at time zero and the wave of mitoses that occurs several hours
later?" As in the discussion of the biochemical events occurring in
continuously dividing cells, the molecular events in which we are

interested here are only those that can be related to the subsequent onset of DNA synthesis and mitosis. While preparing for cell division, the stimulated G_0 cell naturally carries on its fundamental life processes, but since these are not specifically related to cell division, they will be omitted from the present discussion.

With this in mind, let us now turn to the cell populations listed in Tables 5.1 and 5.2 and see what they have taught us, in molecular terms, about the control of cellular proliferation. As mentioned above, any one of these systems has its own special characteristics and its own peculiar problems that can be exploited to gain relevant information, but the fundamental molecular events occurring between the application of the stimulus and the wave of mitoses are substantially the same in all systems studied. There are differences in timing and specific differences due to the nature of the resting cell populations, but the general picture that emerges is very much the same whether quiescent cells are stimulated in culture or in experimental animals. For the sake of clarity, I will describe here in some detail the sequence of biochemical events that occur in the isoproterenol-stimulated salivary gland, but each step or, at least, the most important steps will also be discussed in relation to other systems of stimulated DNA synthesis. The reader is referred to the following review articles for more information on the biochemical events occurring in stimulated G_0 cells: Epifanova and Terskikh (1969) for resting cells in general, Cooper (1971) for phytohemagglutinin-stimulated lymphocytes, Hamilton (1968) for estrogen-stimulated uterus, Epifanova (1971) for estrogens and other hormones, Baserga et al. (1971) for stationary cultures stimulated to proliferate by nutritional changes, and Bucher (1967a,b) for the regenerating liver after partial hepatectomy.

FROM MITOSIS BACKWARD

The stimulation of salivary glands of rodents by isoproterenol was first described by Barka in 1965. The basic experiment is of elegant simplicity. A single injection of isoproterenol, a syn-

TABLE 5.1   Stimulation of Cell Proliferation in Quiescent Cells in Culture

Target cells or tissues	Stimulus	Reference
Stationary cell cultures (3T3)	Nutritional changes	Todaro et al. (1965)
(WI-38)		Wiebel and Baserga (1969)
(3T6)		Salas and Green (1971)
(C3H2K)		Yoshikura and Hirokawa (1968)
(BSC$_1$)		Becker and Levitt (1968)
(BHK21/13)		Burk (1970)
	DNA oncogenic viruses (polyoma)	Dulbecco et al. (1965)
	(SV-40)	Sauer and Defendi (1966)
	(adenovirus)	Zimmerman and Raska (1972)
	Friend leukemia virus	Gabelman et al. (1974)
	Rous sarcoma virus	Macieira-Coelho and Ponten (1967)
	Trypsin	Burger (1970)
Lymphocytes	Phytohemagglutinin	Nowell (1960), Cooper (1971)
	Concanavalin A	Powell and Leon (1970)
	Lima bean lectins	Ruddon et al. (1974)
	Na I O$_4$	Zatz et al. (1972)
	Zn^{++}	Berger and Skinner (1974)

Macrophages	Conditioned medium	Virolainen and Defendi (1967)
Macrophages	Cell fusion with transformed fibroblasts	Croce and Koprowski (1974)
Quiescent nuclei	Cell fusion	Harris (1967)
Skin, mammary gland human fibroblasts	Epidermal growth factor	Cohen (1965) Turkington (1969), Hollenberg and Cuatrecasas (1973)
Mouse mammary gland	Hormones	Lockwood et al. (1967)
Chick embryo fibroblasts	MSA polypeptide	Dulak and Temin (1973)
	Insulin	Vaheri et al. (1973)
	Neuraminidase	Vaheri et al. (1973)
	Trypsin	Vaheri et al. (1973)
	Papain	Vaheri et al. (1973)
Human glia cells	Serum	Ponten et al. (1969)
Serum-deprived chick fibroblasts	Zn^{++}, Mn^{++}, Cd^{++}	Rubin and Koide (1973)
Rabbit kidney cells	Explantation	Lieberman et al. (1963)
Chinese hamster cells	Isoleucine	Tobey and Ley (1970)

TABLE 5.2   Stimulation of Cell Proliferation in Quiescent Cells in Vivo

Target tissue (animal)	Stimulus	Reference
Liver (rat, mouse)	Partial hepatectomy	Grisham (1962), Bucher (1967a,b)
Uterus (rat, mouse)	Estrogens	Hamilton (1968), Epifanova (1971)
Salivary glands (rat, mouse)	Isoproterenol	Barka (1965a), Baserga (1970)
Kidney (rat)	Folic acid	Taylor et al. (1966)
Kidney (rat, mouse)	Controlateral nephrectomy	Malt and Stoddard (1966)
Kidney (rat)	Lead acetate	Choie and Richter (1972)
Mammary gland (mouse)	Estrogens	Bresciani (1971)
Growth cartilage (rat)	Growth hormone	Kember (1971)
Skin (mouse)	Croton oil	Hennings and Boutwell (1970)
	Ethylphenylpropiolate	Raick and Burdzy (1973)
Spleen (mouse)	Erthropoietin	Hodgson (1967)
Adrenal glands (guinea pigs)	ACTH	Masui and Garren (1970)
Liver (rat)	Triiodothyronine	Lee et al. (1968)
Pancreas (rat)	Ethionine	Fitzgerald et al. (1968)
Prostate (castrated rat)	5-α-dihydrotestosterone	Lesser and Bruchovsky (1973)
Liver (fasted rats)	High-protein diet	Short et al. (1973)
Mammary gland (rabbit)	Prolactin	Bourne et al. (1974)
Liver	Albumin depletion	Hill and Saunders (1971)
Pancreas (mouse)	Glucagon + T_3	Malamud and Perrin (1974)

thetic catecholamine (Fig. 5.1), causes, after a lag period of about 20 hours, a marked increase in DNA synthesis in the salivary glands of either rats (Barka 1965a) or mice (Baserga 1970). The increase in DNA synthesis, which reaches a peak about 28 hours after isoproterenol, is followed by a wave of mitoses. In a typical experiment mice are injected intraperitoneally with 0.4 μmol/g body weight of isoproterenol. Thirty hours later, both parotids and submandibular glands contain numerous mitoses, which are exceedingly infrequent in nonstimulated salivary glands of adult rodents. In the parotid, between 60% and 80% of the acinar cells are stimulated to divide by a single injection of isoproterenol.

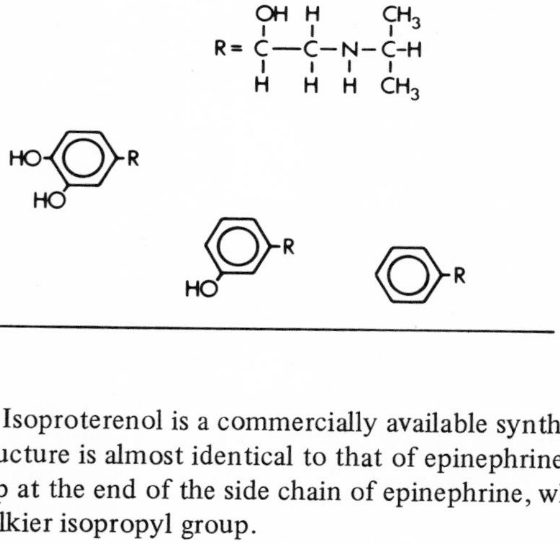

FIGURE 5.1   Isoproterenol is a commercially available synthetic catecholamine whose structure is almost identical to that of epinephrine, except for the methyl group at the end of the side chain of epinephrine, which has been replaced by a bulkier isopropyl group.

In trying to answer the question: "What is the sequence of metabolic events occurring between the administration of isoproterenol and the burst of mitoses?" we shall proceed backward, that is, we shall start from mitosis, the end point, and from there retrace our steps backward to the early chemical events that from a remote distance control mitosis in salivary gland cells.

DNA SYNTHESIS

The first step in our homeward journey is simple. Several years ago Nygaard and Rusch (1955) and Hecht and Van Potter (1956) showed that cell division in regenerating liver is preceded by DNA synthesis, that is, by replication of the genetic material so that the amount of DNA per cell remains constant. It is now well established and, in fact, it is part of the definition of a G_0 cell, as mentioned above, that mitosis in stimulated cells is preceded by replication of DNA. In the isoproterenol stimulated parotid gland, for instance, DNA synthesis begins to increase 20 hours after a single injection of isoproterenol, reaches a peak at about 28-30 hours, and by 42 hours it has returned to control levels. Mitoses, instead, begin to increase in number at about 26 hours, reach a peak between 32-34 hours, and by 48 hours they have returned to control levels (Baserga 1970). As in continuously dividing cells, there is a G_2 period between completion of DNA replication and mitosis. The G_2 period of stimulated G_0 cells is indistinguishable from that of continuously dividing cells, and the reader is referred to chapter 3 for the biochemical events occurring during the G_2 phase. Similarly, the reader is referred to Chapter 2 for the biochemistry of the S phase, which is the same in continuously dividing cells and in stimulated G_0 cells. I shall limit myself to point out that the synthesis of histones, as in continuously dividing cells, has been shown to occur exclusively in the S phase, both in the isoproterenol-stimulated salivary glands (Baserga 1970) and regenerating liver after partial hepatectomy (Takai et al. 1968).

At the time of onset of DNA synthesis, centrioles commence replication (Robbins et al. 1968), and at the same time, or just before it, a number of enzymes that are related to DNA synthesis increase in activity or make their de novo apprearance. Four such enzymes have been studied in some detail in the isoproterenol-stimulated salivary gland of mice. Thymidine kinase and thymidylate kinase begin to increase at about 20 hours after isoproterenol, reaching a peak at about the same time as the DNA synthesis peak (Pegoraro and Baserga 1970). Thymidylate synthetase and DNA polymerase, instead, increase at about 18 hours before isoproterenol, that is, about 2 hours before the onset of DNA synthesis. DNA polymerase activity returns to control levels, like DNA synthesis, by 48 hours (Barka 1965b), while thymidylate synthetase remains elevated even 48 hours after isoproterenol, another example showing the lack of synchrony between the activities of enzymes connected with DNA synthesis and the synthesis of DNA itself. As discussed in Chapter 2, the increased activity of enzymes related to DNA synthesis or the increased concentration of deoxynucleotide triphosphates are the favorite topic of debutantes in the field of cell proliferation, and these two parameters have been studied in almost every population of stimulated G_0 cells. In general, enzymes and precursors begin to increase at the time DNA synthesis begins to increase and remain elevated even when DNA synthesis has returned to control levels. For instance, in regenerating liver the concentration of deoxythymidine triphosphate begins to increase at the time of the increase in DNA synthesis, but remains elevated even 45 hours after partial hepatectomy when DNA synthesis has all but ceased (Bucher and Oakman 1969). Other examples have been given in chapter 2. More important that the intracellular concentration of deoxynucleotides is the observation that, coincidentally with the onset of DNA synthesis, there is, in stimulated 3T3 cells, an increase in the uptake of thymidine and deoxycitidine (Cunningham and Remo 1973). Since the uptake of purine deoxynucleosides or orthophosphate is not affected, this change could reflect a specific alteration of membrane function at the time of DNA synthesis.

THE LATE PREREPLICATIVE PHASE

The time of appearance of the templates coding for thymidine kinase, thymidylate kinase and thymidylate synthetase, has been determined in the isoproterenol-stimulated parotid gland of mice by Pegoraro and Baserga (1970). These authors injected actinomycin D at varying intervals after isoproterenol and then measured enzyme activity at 28 hours, the peak of activity for all three enzymes. When actinomycin D was injected at 18 hours or later, after the administration of isoproterenol, enzyme activity at 28 hours was the same as in isoproterenol-stimulated salivary glands of mice not injected with actinomycin D. However, if actinomycin D was injected at any time during the first 12 hours after isoproterenol, enzyme activity at 28 hours remained at the levels of control mice not injected with isoproterenol. Between 12 and 18 hours the effect of actinomycin D was intermediate. The results indicated that the synthesis of the RNA templates coding for these three enzymes was completed by the 18th hour after isoproterenol injection. An obvious objection to this kind of experiment is that actinomycin D may exert generalized toxic effects on cells, which become apparent only after a certain number of hours. However, the isoproterenol-stimulated salivary glands offer a built-in control. Immediately after the administration of isoproterenol, the salivary glands secrete copiously and the extent of secretion can easily be measured by determining the α-amylase activity of the gland. Within 2 hours after the administration of isoproterenol, α-amylase activity has decreased to about 10% of control values. Beginning at 12 hours after isoproterenol, αamylase activity increases again due to new enzyme synthesis (Byrt 1966) and by 24 hours it has returned to the level of control glands from animals not injected with isoproterenol. When actinomycin D is given in large doses to isoproterenol-stimulated mice, the decrease in α-amylase activity and its return to control levels continue unperturbed. In other words, it seems that after actinomycin D the salivary glands are capable of continuing protein synthesis at a normal rate. If actinomycin D can inhibit the appearance of certain enzymes, it seems reasonable to assume that it is not due to a generalized toxic effect, but to some more specific effect preceding the translational process.

Continuing our journey backward from mitosis, we find two important events occurring between 8 and 12 hours after isoproterenol. The first is an increase in protein synthesis that reaches a peak in stimulated salivary glands 8 hours after isoproterenol (Sasaki et al. 1969). This increased protein synthesis in the middle of the prereplicative phase has been reported in other G_0 cells stimulated to proliferate (see some of the reviews cited in Tables 5.1 and 5.2 for further information). Occasionally, the synthesis of certain specific proteins is markedly enhanced a few hours before DNA synthesis, as albumin in regenerating liver (Majumdar et al. 1967) or transferrin in phytohemagglutinin-stimulated lymphocytes (Tormey and Mueller 1972).

A second important event occurring at about this time is a peak in the synthesis of cytoplasmic ribosomal RNA, both 18S and 28S. The incorporation of [^{3}H]-uridine into cytoplasmic ribosomal RNA of salivary glands reaches a peak between 8 and 12 hours after isoproterenol. This is not due to a change in pool size since the increase in uridine incorporation into total cellular RNA is fivefold above control levels, while the increase in uridine incorporation into cytoplasmic ribosomal RNA is elevenfold above control levels (Novi and Baserga 1972). An increased synthesis of ribosomal RNA has been known for some time to be a prerequisite for cell growth (Tata 1968, 1970), and accordingly it has been reported in many situations in which quiescent cells have been stimulated to proliferate from stationary cells stimulated by nutritional changes (Lieberman et al. 1963, Ellem and Mironescu 1972, Zardi and Baserga 1974) to the regenerating liver (Fujioka et al. 1963), and from phytohemagglutinin-stimulated lymphocytes (Cooper 1971) to the estrogen-stimulated uterus (Hamilton 1968, Epifanova 1971). The synthesis of ribosomal RNA actually begins to increase early in the prereplicative phase (Chaudhuri et al. 1967, Cooper 1971, Maniatis et al. 1973, Zardi and Baserga 1974) and, in fact, according to Mauck and Green (1973) the synthesis of ribosomal RNA begins to increase within 10 minutes after quiescent 3T6 cells are stimulated to proliferate. This early increase will be discussed further, later. For the moment, let us say that the peak of ribosomal RNA synthesis is usually reached in the middle of the lag phase, and that it can be used to conveniently divide the prereplicative phase into early and late.

The question may arise whether the various events that have been described thus far are related, or not, to the subsequent onset of DNA synthesis and cell division. Again, the isoproterenol-stimulated salivary gland offers an excellent built-in control. This is due to the peculiarity of the stimulus, which is apparently very brief (Baserga 1970). Thus, if xycloheximide in the amount of 33 μg/g body weight is injected into mice 1 hour after isoproterenol, the subsequent increases in DNA synthesis at 20 hours and mitoses at 28 hours are effectively suppressed. This is not due to a direct toxic action of cycloheximide since, at this dosage, cycloheximide inhibits protein synthesis in mouse salivary glands for only a brief period of 2 hours (Sasaki et al. 1969). In fact, cycloheximide has an inhibitory effect on the subsequent increase in DNA synthesis only when injected between 1 and 6 hours after isoproterenol: at 12 hours, it has no effect whatsoever (Novi and Baserga 1972). Furthermore, when cycloheximide is given 1 hour after isoproterenol, it does not interfere with the resynthesis of α-amylase at later hours, but several events, including the increase in protein synthesis at 8 hours and the peak of cytoplasmic ribosomal RNA synthesis between 8 and 12 hours, are permanently suppressed (Novi and Baserga 1972). It seems, therefore, that if one inhibits protein synthesis in salivary glands for 2 hours early in the pre-replicative phase, the whole chain of biochemical events that leads to the onset of DNA synthesis is permanently interrupted. This is more difficult to obtain in other systems as, for instance, regenerating liver after partial hepatectomy. The stimulus (the liver stump) persists even after the biochemical processes have been interrupted by inhibitors, and the persistance of the stimulus, when the effect of inhibitors wears off, eventually causes regeneration to take place.

We have mentioned above that the peak of ribosomal RNA synthesis divides the lag period between the stimulus and DNA synthesis into an early phase and late prereplicative phase. The decision to chose the peak of cytoplasmic ribosomal RNA synthesis as the dividing line is essentially arbitrary. It has a weak foundation on the observation that, when the lag period between the administration of isoproterenol and DNA synthesis is shortened by appropriate manipulations, the peak of cytoplasmic ribosomal RNA synthesis remains at a constant distance from the onset of DNA synthesis (Novi and Baserga 1972). If confirmed in other systems, it would suggest that the prereplicative phase can be divided into two parts: an early part of variable length and a late part of fixed length.

THE EARLY PREREPLICATIVE PHASE

A number of biochemical markers have been described in the early prereplicative phase of cells stimulated to proliferate that can reasonably be considered related to the subsequent stimulation of DNA synthesis and cell division. Three biochemical processes that are of paramount importance, namely: (a) the changes occurring on the cell surface; (b) the activation of the genome; and (c) the increased synthesis of nonhistone chromosomal proteins will be discussed in detail in subsequent chapters. I shall discuss here other presumably important early events occurring in stimulated cells, but first let me illustrate again how the isoproterenol-stimulated salivary gland can be exploited to investigate the relationship of a given biochemical event to the subsequent stimulation of cell proliferation. As already mentioned, isoproterenol is a synthetic catecholamine which has essentially the same structure as epinephrine, except that the methyl group at the end of the side chain has been replaced by a bulkier isopropyl group (Fig. 5.1). There is an analog of isoproterenol, 1-phenyl-2-isopropylaminoethanol, which resembles isoproterenol in all respects except that the two hydroxyl groups on the phenyl ring are missing. When 1-phenyl-2-isopropylaminoethanol is injected, dissolved in 0.1 N HCl, into a mouse, it is hydroxylated and it becomes isoproterenol (Labows et al. 1971). However, when 1-phenyl-2-isopropylaminoethanol is injected, dissolved in 40% ethanol, it is not hydroxylated. In both cases the isoproterenol analog causes a marked stimulation of secretion, but only when injected after it is dissolved in 0.1 N HCl, and therefore hydroxylated, is 1-phenyl-2-isopropylaminoethanol capable of stimulating DNA synthesis in mouse parotids. It is therefore possible, using this analog, to determine which events are related to secretion and which are related to DNA synthesis and cell division. For instance, an event of certainly considerable importance that occurs in the early prereplicative phase is an increase in the rate of synthesis of nonhistone chromosomal proteins. Stein and Baserga (1970) have shown that the synthesis of nonhistone chromosomal proteins increases markedly between 30 minutes and 12 hours after a single administration of isoproterenol. Baserga and Stein (1971) have also shown that the stimulation of synthesis of nonhistone chromosomal proteins occurs also with 1-phenyl-2-isopropylaminoethanol dissolved in 0.1 N HCl, but that there is no increase when the isoproterenol analog is injected after it is dissolved in 40% ethanol (ethanol has no effect on the stimulation caused by isoproterenol itself). Similarly, the increase in the synthesis of cytoplasmic ribosomal RNA occurs when the analog is injected dissolved in 0.1 N HCl but not when it is dissolved in 40% ethanol before it is injected (Novi and Baserga 1972).

FROM CYCLIC NUCLEOTIDES TO POLYAMINES

When density inhibited confluent monolayers of 3T3 cells are stimulated to proliferate by trypsin, there is a prompt decrease in the amount of intracellular cyclic AMP (Burger et al. 1972). The level of cyclic AMP then increases again and remains elevated during S phase, to drop again at mitosis. Several proteases that stimulate cell proliferation in rodent cells cause a decrease in cAMP levels. Furthermore, dibutyril-cAMP (at a concentration of 10^{-4} M) inhibits growth stimulation by either serum or pronase (Bombik and Burger 1973). Essentially similar results have been obtained in human diploid fibroblasts (stimulated by serum) by Froehlich and Rachmeler (1972). These studies, indicating a cAMP-sensitive step in the early prereplicative phase of cells stimulated to proliferate, are the logical conclusion of an avalanche of papers that have popularized the theory of cAMP as a regulator, indeed, as *the* regulator of cell growth. Most of these studies are based on two different but related observations, namely: (a) intracellular cAMP levels are low in transformed and growing untransformed cells and high in stationary cell cultures (Heidrick and Ryan 1971, Sheppard 1972, Pastan et al. 1974) and (b) addition of cAMP to culture medium inhibits the growth of cells (Johnson et al. 1971, Sheppard 1971). While there is no question that the evidence for an inhibitory effect of cAMP on cell proliferation is substantial, the results are by no means unanimous. To begin with, isoproterenol causes an immediate and dramatic increase in intracellular levels of cAMP in the stimulated salivary gland (Durham et al. 1974) and, although it is true that we can rationalize anything we wish to rationalize, this heretical finding has not yet been explained. In BHK21 cells, according to Zimmerman and Raska (1972), dibutyril-cAMP inhibits DNA synthesis induced by adenovirus type 12 but not DNA synthesis induced by a nutritional change. Even more confusing are the results of Oey et al. (1974) using cell lines that stop growing either by contact-inhibition (density-revertants) or by serum depletion (serum-revertants). A marked increase in cAMP intracellular concentration occurred only in serum-depleted cultures of serum-revertants. Density-dependent inhibition of growth was not accompanied by an increase in cAMP concentration. Similar results were obtained by Seifert and Paul (1972) and by Burstin et al (1974), the latter using SV-40 transformed cell lines that were temperature-sensitive for growth. Finally, at least in the case of polyoma-transformed 3T3 cells (Py 3T3), the inhibitory effect of dibutyril-cAMP on cell growth is much delayed in comparison to membrane changes, and Py 3T3 cells undergo more than two doublings in cell number before succumbing to the effect of cAMP (Grimes and Schroder 1973).

As the fortunes of cAMP began to decline, another cyclic nucleotide made its appearance on the horizon of cell proliferation; cyclic GMP (Goldberg et al. 1974, Estensen et al. 1974). Stimulation of lymphocytes by phytohemagglutinin causes a marked increase in cGMP (Hadden et al. 1972) and cyclic GMP or its derivatives stimulate DNA synthesis in quiescent 3T3 cells (Siefert and Rudland 1974). The stimulation, however, is much lower than that caused by fresh serum. Intracellular concentration of cGMP is also increased in 3T3 cells and lymphocytes stimulated to proliferate by the tumor promoter, phorbol myristate acetate (Estensen et al. 1974). Actually, the data of Goldberg et al. (1974) and Estensen et al. (1974) seem to disprove rather than support a role of cGMP in cell proliferation. In the systems studied, the entry of cells into DNA synthesis is somewhat asynchronous, an interval of 6 or more hours elapsing between the first and the last cells entering S. Yet, the increase in cGMP concentration lasts for only 45 seconds early after stimulation. If cGMP were truly correlated to the subsequent entry of cells into S phase, its increase should be sustained longer or the entrance of cells into S should be more synchronous, a dilemma that has also been perceived by Green (1974) in relation to cAMP. It is hard to say at this point how important cyclic nucleotides are in the regulation of cell proliferation. Undoubtedly, they have a role, stimulatory for cGMP, inhibitory for cAMP, at least in some cells. Further studies will have to decide the specificity of changes in intracellular concentrations and whether they are the cause or the effect of the stimulation to proliferate. Perhaps their role is to mediate the phosphorylation of critical nuclear proteins. While this topic will be considered in more detail in chapter 7, I shall mention here that the activity of chromatin-bound protein kinases is known to increase in two situations in which quiescent cells are stimulated to proliferate, the salivary glands after isoproterenol (Ishida and Ahmed 1974) and the folic-acid stimulated kidney (Brade et al. 1974).

Leaving cyclic nucleotides aside for the moment, let us look at another event occurring during the early prereplicative phase and apparently related to cell growth, namely the increase in the intracellular concentration of polyamines (putrescine, spermine and spermidine) and of some enzymes connected with their metabolism. An increase in intracellular content of polyamines and in the activity of two related enzymes, L-ornithine decarboxylase and S-adenosyl-L-methionine decarboxylase, has been reported in several situations in which quiescent cells are stimulated to proliferate, including regenerating liver after partial hepatectomy (Russell and Snyder 1968, Raina et al. 1966), estrogen-stimulated uterus, (Russell and Taylor 1971), androgen-stimulated prostate (Pegg et al. 1970), and lymphocytes stimulated by phytohemagglutinin (Kay and Lindsay 1973). In regenerating liver the activity of ornithine decarboxylase is tripled within 1 hour after partial hepatectomy and reaches a peak at 16 hours, when it is twenty-fivefold above control levels (Russell and Snyder 1968). The increase correlates with stimulation of cell proliferation (Gaza et al. 1973). In WI-38 fibroblasts stimulated to proliferate by a nutritional change, the increase in polyamines seems to correlate with the synthesis of ribosomal RNA (Heby et al 1974), a finding which agrees with two other observations: (a) polyamines are most often localized in the ribosomal fraction of rat liver (Raina and Telaranta 1967), and (b) the cellular content of putrescine, spermidine, and spermine doubles from G_1 to mitosis (Heby et al. 1973), together with the doubling of ribosomal RNA.

The reader may find more detailed information on polyamines and growth in a recent book (Russell 1973). From our point of view we may say that, like cyclic nucleotides, polyamines certainly have a role in cell growth, but what their role is, is not yet clear (Harik et al. 1974).

A GENERAL VIEW OF THE PREREPLICATIVE PHASE

Our present knowledge of the sequence of biochemical events occurring from the application of the stimulus to mitosis is summarized in Fig. 5.2. As mentioned above, gene activation itself and the phenomena accompanying and preceding gene activation will be discussed in subsequent chapters. At this point we will pause to make some reflections on the sequence of biochemical events that follow gene activation.

A few important things should be noticed from Fig. 5.2, (a) gene activation occurs early in the prereplicative phase, (b) there are events that accompany and precede gene activation, (c) after gene activation there is an alternation of RNA and protein synthesis in a ping-pong mechanism in which a round of protein synthesis is

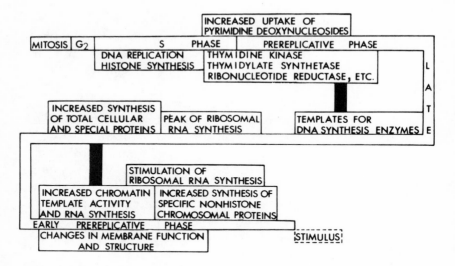

FIGURE 5.2   Plato's universal G_0 cell stimulated to proliferate.

preceded by RNA synthesis and precedes, in turn, another round
of RNA synthesis. This would indicate, in stimulated G_0 cells, a
sequential gene activation similar to the one described in yeast
cells prior to DNA synthesis (Hereford and Hartwell 1974). However, in our discussion I shall restrict the term *gene activation* to
the *initial* increase in gene activity (see chapter 6). (d) The ping-
pong mechanism just mentioned is reminiscent of a similar sequence of events occurring during the transcription of the genome
of T4 and T7 phages in which the products of early RNA molecules are necessary for the synthesis of late RNA molecules (Salser
et al. 1970). A ping-pong, or cascading mechanism for sequential
gene activation has also been reported in salivary gland chromosomes of *Chironomus tentans* by Clever (1964), in salivary gland
chromosomes of *Drosophia melanogaster* by Ashburner (1973),
and in germinating wheat by Dobrzanska et al. (1973). This mechanism is further supported by the findings of Church and McCarthy
(1967) who investigated, by RNA/DNA hybridization techniques,
the species of RNA synthesized in mouse liver before and after

partial hepatectomy. Church and McCarthy showed that the RNA species made at 1 and 3 hours after partial hepatectomy differ from each other. RNA species made at 6 and 12 hours differ from those made at 1 or 3 hours and from each other, as well as from the RNA species that are made in normal quiescent mouse liver. The conclusions of Church and McCarthy (1967) are valid, although the hybridization techniques used detected, in all probability, only repetitive sequences. They indicate that the repetitive sequences transcribed by regenerating liver vary with time after partial hepatectomy. The importance of these findings cannot be considered trivial in view of the fact that repetitive sequences, especially middle-repetitive sequences, are interspersed with single-copy sequences in nuclear RNA (Holmes and Bonner 1974) and are found, reduced in size, even in polysomal messenger RNA (Firtel and Lodish 1973, Dina et al. 1974). A ping-pong mechanism is also present in 3T3 cells stimulated to proliferate by pronase. The stimulation can be inhibited by actinomycin D only between 0-1 hour and 4-5 hours after treatment, while protein synthesis is required only between 1-2 and 4-5 hours after pronase (Noonan and Burger 1973). We have seen before that cycloheximide inhibits isoproterenol-stimulated DNA synthesis only when given between 0 and 6 hours after the stimulus. It seems that after a few hours, the stimulated cell is committed to DNA synthesis, perhaps through the stabilization of messenger RNA (Buckingham et al. 1974). (e) Ribosomal RNA synthesis almost invariably precedes DNA synthesis independently of the synthesis of new species of messenger RNA. (f) There is a considerable interval between the application of the stimulus and the onset of DNA synthesis, and yet this interval is filled with many biochemical events whose relatedness to DNA synthesis and cell division can be supported by adequate controls and correlations.

These biochemical markers have been consistently found in many situations in which quiescent cells are stimulated to proliferate. I shall mention here, very briefly, one system because it will be studied in detail in subsequent chapters. In confluent monolayers of WI-38 human diploid fibroblasts stimulated to proliferate by nutritional changes, RNA and protein synthesis are also increased. In a typical experiment, WI-38 fibroblasts are left to grow in the original medium in which they were plated, and under these conditions, when they reach a confluent monolayer, usually by the 5th day after plating, they stop dividing. When the medium is replaced by fresh medium containing 10%-30% fetal calf serum, from 60% to 80% of the quiescent cells are stimulated to synthesize DNA and divide (Baserga et al. 1971). The interval between the change of medium and the increase in DNA synthesis is 12-15 hours (Farber et al. 1971), and RNA synthesis increases within 1 hour after the change of medium. The increased RNA synthesis will be discussed further in chapter 6, while in chapter 7 we shall discuss the increase in the synthesis of nonhistone chromosomal proteins that also occurs promptly after WI-38 cells are stimulated to proliferate by a change of medium.

A few words, finally, on the possibility of a two-step mechanism in the stimulation of DNA synthesis and cell division. A number of investigators have suggested in one way or another that more than one step is required for the orderly flow of G_0 cells into DNA synthesis and cell division. It can be demonstrated, for instance, that the addition of serum is essential only for the stimulation of quiescent cells and that, after the cells have been properly stimulated, serum can be removed without interrupting the flow of cells from G_0 to S (Burk 1970, Temin 1971). However, the question is not whether there are two steps or one single step, but whether there are two steps or several steps, as shown in the present chapter.

In conclusion a picture emerges that after the application of a proliferative stimulus, a series of biochemical events occurs that eventually leads to the onset of DNA synthesis and finally to mitosis. As mentioned above, a possible critical step in triggering the sequence of events is the activation of the genome. The evidence for genome activation will be the subject of our discussion in the next chapter.

REFERENCES

Armstrong, R. L. and Sueoka, N. (1968). *Proc. Natl. Acad. Sci. USA 59:* 153-160.

Ashburner, M. (1973). *Develop. Biol. 35:* 47-61.

Barka, T. (1965a). *Exp. Cell Res. 39:* 355-364.

Barka, T. (1965b). *Exp. Cell Res. 37:* 662-679.

Baserga, R. (1968). *Cell Tissue Kinet. 1:* 167-191.

Baserga, R. (1970). Control of DNA Synthesis in Mammalian Cells. Miami Winter Symposia, North Holland Publ. Co. Amsterdam, 2, pp. 447-461.

Baserga, R. Rovera, G., and Farber, J. (1971). *In Vitro 7:* 80-87.

Baserga, R. and Stein, G. (1971). *Fed. Proc. 30:* 1752-1759.

Becker, Y. and Levitt, J. (1968). *Exp. Cell Res. 51:* 27-33.

Berger, N. A. and Skinner, A. M. (1974). *J. Cell Biol. 61:* 45-55.

Bombik, B. M. and Burger, M. M. (1973). *Exp. Cell Res. 80:* 88-94.

Bourne, R. A., Bryant, J. A., and Falconer, I. R. (1974). *J. Cell Sci. 14:* 105-111.

Brade, W. P., Thomson, J. A., Chiu, J. F., and Hnilica, L. S. (1974). *Exp. Cell Res. 84:* 183-190.

Bresciani, F. (1971). Ovarian Steroid Control of Cell Proliferation in Mammary Gland Cancer. In *Basic Actions of Sex Steroids on Target Organs.* S. Karger, Basel, pp. 130-159.

Bucher, N. L. R. (1967a). *N. Engl. J. Med. 277:* 686-696.

Bucher, N. L. R. (1967b). *N. Engl. J. Med. 277:* 738-746.

Bucher, N. L. R. and Oakman, N. J. (1969). *Biochim. Biophys. Acta 186:* 13-20.

Buckingham, M. E., Caput, D., Cohen, A., Whalen, R. G., and Gros, F. (1974). *Proc. Natl. Acad. Sci. 71:* 1466-1470.

Burger, M. M. (1970). *Nature 227:* 170-171.

Burger, M. M., Bombik, B. M., Breckenridge, B. M., and Sheppard, J. R. (1972). *Nature New Biol. 239:* 161-163.

Burk, R. R. (1970). *Exp. Cell Res 63:* 309-316.

Burstin, S. J., Renger, H. C., and Basilico, C. (1974). *J. Cell Physiol. 84:* 69-73.

Byrt, P. (1966). *Nature 212:* 1212-1215.

Chaudhuri, S., Doi, O., and Lieberman, I. (1967). *Biochim. Biophys. Acta 134:* 479-480.

Choie, D. D. and Richter, G. W. (1972). *Am. J. Pathol. 66:* 265-275.

Church, R. B. and McCarthy, B. J. (1967). *J. Mol. Biol. 23:* 459-475.

Clever, U. (1964). *Science 146:* 794-795.

Cohen, S. (1965). *Develop. Biol. 12:* 394-407.

Cooper, H. L. (1971). Biochemical Alterations Accompanying Initiation of Growth in Resting Cells. In *The Cell Cycle and Cancer*, R. Baserga (Ed.). Marcel Dekker, New York, pp. 197-226.

Croce, C. M., and Koprowski, H. (1974). *J. Exptl. Med. 139:* 1350-1353.

Cunningham, D. D. and Remo, R. A. (1973). *J. Biol. Chem. 248:*6282-6288.

Dina, D., Meza, I., and Crippa, M. (1974). *Nature 248:* 486-490.

Dobrzanska, M., Tomaszewski; M., Grzelczak, S., Rejman. E., and Buchowicz, J. (1973). *Nature 244:* 507-508.

Dulak, N. C. and Temin, H. M. (1973). *J. Cell. Physiol. 81:* 153-160.

Dulbecco, R., Hartwell, L. H., and Vogt, M. (1965). *Proc. Natl. Acad. Sci. USA 53:* 403-410.

Durham, J. P., Baserga, R., and Butcher, F. R. (1974). In *Control of Proliferation in Animal Cells*, B. Clarkson and R. Baserga (Eds.). Cold Spring Harbor, pp. 595-607.

Ellem, K. A. O. and Mironescu, S. (1972). *J. Cell Physiol. 79:* 389-406.

Epifanova, O. I. (1971). Effects of Hormones on the Cell Cycle. In *The Cell Cycle and Cancer*, R. Baserga (Ed.). Marcel Dekker, New York, pp. 197-226.

Epifanova, O. I. and Terskikh, V. V. (1969). *Cell Tissue Kinet. 2:* 75-93.

Estensen, R. D., Hadden, J. W., Hadden, E. M., Touraine, F., Touraine, J., Haddox, M. K., and Goldberg, N. D. (1974). In *Control of Proliferation in Animal Cells,* B. Clarkson and R. Baserga (Eds.). Cold Spring Harbor, pp. 627-634.

Farber, J., Rovera, G., and Baserga, R. (1971). *Biochem. J. 122:* 189-195.

Firtel, R. A. and Lodish, H. F. (1973). *J. Mol. Biol. 79:* 295-314.

Fitzgerald, P. G., Herman, L., Carol, B., Rogue, A., Marsh, W. H., Rosenstock, L., and Richards, C. (1968). *Am. J. Pathol. 52:* 983-1012.

Froehlich, J. E. and Rachmeler, M. (1972). *J. Cell. Biol. 55:* 19-31.

Fujioka, M., Koga, M., and Lieberman, I. (1963). *J. Biol. Chem. 238:* 3401-3406.

Gabelman, N., Scher, W., and Friend, C. (1974). *Int. J. Cancer 13:* 343-352.

Gaza, D. J., Short, J., and Lieberman, I. (1973). *FEBS Letters 32:* 251-253.

Goldberg, N. D., Haddox, M. K., Dunham, E., Lopez, C., and Hadden, J. W. (1974). In *Control of Proliferation in Animal Cells*, B. Clarkson and R. Baserga (Eds.). Cold Spring Harbor, pp. 609-625.

Green, H. (1974). In *Control of Proliferation in Animal Cells*, B. Clarkson and R. Baserga (Eds.). Cold Spring Harbor Laboratory, pp. 743-755.

Grimes, W. J. and Schroeder, J. L. (1973). *J. Cell Biol. 56:* 487-491.

Grisham, J. W. (1962). *Cancer Res. 22:* 842-849.

Hadden, J. W., Hadden, E. M., Haddox, M. K., and Goldberg, N. D. (1972). *Proc. Natl. Acad. Sci. USA 69:* 3024-3027.

Hamilton, T. H. (1968). *Science 161:* 649-661.

Harik, S. I., Hollenberg, M. D., and Snyder, S. H. (1974). *Nature 249:* 250-251.

Harris, H. J. (1967). *J. Cell Sci. 2:* 23-32.

Heby, O., Marton, L. J., Zardi, L., Russell, D. H., and Baserga, R. (1974). In *The Cell Cycle in Malignancy and Immunity*, AEC Symposium Series.

Heby, O., Sarna, G. P., Marton, L. J., Omine, M., Perry, S., and Russell, D. H. (1973). *Cancer Res. 33:* 2959-2964.

Hecht, L. I. and Van Potter, V. R. (1956). *Cancer Res. 16:* 988-993.

Heidrick, M. L. and Ryan, W. L. (1971). *Cancer Res. 31:* 1313-1315.

Hennings, H. and Boutwell, R. K. (1970). *Cancer Res. 30:* 312-320.

Hereford, L. M. and Hartwell, L. H. (1974). *J. Mol. Biol. 84:* 445-461.

Hill, B. and Saunders, E. H. (1971). *Lab. Invest. 24:* 325-330.

Hodgson, G. (1967). *Proc. Soc. Exp. Biol. Med. 124:* 1045-1047.

Hollenberg, M. D. and Cuatrecasas, P. (1973). *Proc. Natl. Acad. Sci. USA 70:* 2964-2968.

Holmes, D. S. and Bonner, J. (1974). *Proc. Natl. Acad. Sci. 71:* 1108-1112.

Ishida, H. and Ahmed, K. (1974). *Exp. Cell Res. 84:* 127-136.

Johnson, G. S., Friedman, R. M., and Pastan, I. (1971). *Proc. Natl. Acad. Sci. USA 68:* 425-429.

Kay, J. E. and Lindsay, V. J. (1973). *Exp. Cell Res. 77:* 428-436.

Kember, N. F. (1971). *Cell Tissue Kinet. 4:* 193-199.

Kobayashi, Y., Steinberg, W., Higa, A., Halvorson, H. O., and Levinthal, C. (1965). In *Spores III*, L. L. Campbell and H. O. Halvorson (Eds.). Am. Soc. for Microbiology, Ann Arbor, Mich. pp. 200-212.

Labows, J., Swern, D., and Baserga, R. (1971). *Chemico-Biol. Interactions 3:* 449-457.

Lee, K., Sun, S., and Miller, O. H. (1968). *Arch. Biochem. Biophys. 125:* 751-757.

Lesser, B. and Bruchovsky, N. (1973). *Biochim. Biophys. Acta 308:* 426-437.

Lieberman, I., Abrams, R., and Ove, P. (1963). *J. Biol. Chem. 238:* 2141-2149.

Lockwood, D. H., Stockdale, F. E., Topper, Y. J. (1967). *Science 156:* 945-946.

Macieira-Coelho, A. and Ponten, J. (1967). *Biochem. Biophys. Res. Comm. 29:* 316-321.

Majumdar, C., Tsukada, K., and Lieberman, I. (1967). *J. Biol. Chem. 242:* 700-704.

Malamud, D. and Perrin, L. (1974). *Endocrinology 94:* 1157-1160.

Malt, R. A. and Stoddard, S. K. (1966). *Biochim. Biophys. Acta 119:* 207-210.

Maniatis, G. M., Rifkind, R. A., Bank, A., and Marks, P. A. (1973). *Proc. Natl. Acad. Sci. 70:* 3189-3194.

Masui, H. and Garren, L. D. (1970). *J. Biol. Chem. 245:* 2627-2632.

Mauck, J. C. and Green, H. (1973). *Proc. Natl. Acad. Sci. USA 70:* 2819-2822.

Noonan, K. D. and Burger, M. M. (1973). *Exp. Cell Res. 80:* 405-414.

Novi. A. M. and Baserga, R. (1972). *Lab. Invest. 26:* 540-547.

Nowell, P. (1960). *Cancer Res. 60:* 462-466.

Nygaard, O. and Rusch, H. P. (1955). *Cancer Res. 15:* 240-245.

Oey, J., Vogel, A., and Pollack, R. (1974). *Proc. Natl. Acad. Sci. USA 71:* 694-698.

Pastan, I., Anderson, W. B., Carchman, R. A., Willingham, M. C., Russell, T. R., and Johnson, G. S. (1974). In *Control of Proliferation in Animal Cells,* B. Clarkson and R. Baserga (Eds.). Cold Spring Harbor, pp. 563-570.

Pegg, A. E., Lockwood, D. H., and Williams-Ashman, H. G. (1970). *Biochem. J. 117:* 17-31.

Pegoraro, L. and Baserga, R. (1970). *Lab. Invest. 22:* 266-271.

Ponten, J., Westermark, B., and Hugosson, R. (1969). *Exp. Cell Res. 58:* 393-400.

Powell, A. E. and Leon, M. A. (1970). *Exp. Cell Res. 62:* 315-325.

Raick, A. N. and Burdzy, K. (1973). *Cancer Res. 33:* 2221-2230.

Raina, A., Janne, J., and Siimes, M. (1966). *Biochim. Biophys. Acta 123:* 197-201.

Raina, A. and Telaranta, T. (1967). *Biochim. Biophys. Acta 138:* 200-203.

Robbins, E., Jentzsch, G., and Micali, A. (1968). *J. Cell Biol. 36:* 329-339.

Rubin, H. and Koide, T. J. (1973). *J. Cell Physiol. 81:* 387-396.

Ruddon, R. W., Weisenthal, L. M., Lundeen, D. E., Bessler, W., and Goldstein, I. J. (1974). *Proc. Natl. Acad. Sci. USA 71:* 1848-1851.

Russell, D. H. (Ed.) (1973). *Polyamines in Normal and Neoplastic Growth.* Raven Press, New York, passim.

Russell, D. H. and Snyder, S. H. (1968). *Proc. Natl. Acad. Sci. USA 60:* 1420-1427.

Russell, D. H. and Taylor, R. L. (1971). *Endocrinology 88:* 1397-1403.

Salas, J. and Green, H. (1971). *Nature New Biol. 229:* 165-169.

Salser, W., Bolle, A. and Epstein, R. (1970). *J. Mol. Biol. 49:* 271-295.

Sasaki, T., Litwack, G. and Baserga, R. (1969). *J. Biol. Chem. 244:* 4831-4837.

Sauer, G. and Defendi, V. (1966). *Proc. Natl. Acad. Sci. USA 56:* 452-457.

Seifert, W. and Paul, D. (1972). *Nature New Biol. 240:* 281-283.

Seifert, W. and Rudland, P. S. (1974). *Nature 248:* 138-140.

Sheppard, J. R. (1971). *Proc. Natl. Acad. Sci. USA 68:* 1316-1320.

Sheppard, J. R. (1972). *Nature New Biol. 236:* 14-16.

Short, J., Armstrong, N. B., Zemel, R., and Lieberman, I. (1973). *Biochem. Biophys. Res. 50:* 430-437.

Stein, G. and Baserga, R. (1970). *J. Biol. Chem. 245:* 6097-6105.

Takai, S., Borun, T., Muchmore, J., and Lieberman, I. (1968). *Nature 219:* 860-861.

Tata, J. R., (1968). *Nature 219:* 331-337.

Tata, J. R., (1970). *Biochem. J. 116:* 617-630.

Taylor, D. M., Threlfall, G., and Buck, A. T. (1966). *Nature 212:* 472-474.

Temin, H. M. (1971). *J. Cell Physiol. 78:* 161-170.

Tobey, R. A. and Ley, K. D. (1970). *J. Cell Biol. 46:* 151-157.

Todaro, G. J., Lazar, G. K., and Green, H. (1965). *J. Cell Comp. Physiol. 66:* 325-333.

Tormey, D. C. and Mueller, G. C. (1972). *Exp. Cell Res. 74:* 220-226.

Turkington, R. W. (1969). *Exp. Cell Res. 57:* 79-85.

Vaheri, A., Ruoslahti, E., Hovi, T., and Nordling, S. (1973). *J. Cell. Physiol. 81:* 355-364.

Virolainen, M. and Defendi, V. (1967). Wistar Inst. Symposium Monogr. No. 7, 67-86.

Wiebel, F. and Baserga, R. (1969). *J. Cell. Physiol. 74:* 191-202.

Yoshikura, H. and Hirokawa, Y. (1968). *Exp. Cell Res. 52:* 439-444.

Zardi, L. and Baserga, R. (1974). *Exp. Mol. Pathol. 20:* 69-77.

Zatz, M. M., Goldstein, A. L., Blumfeld, O. O. and White, A. (1972). *Nature New Biol. 240:* 252-255.

Zimmerman, J. E. Jr. and Raska, K., Jr. (1972). *Nature New Biol. 239:* 145-147.

SIX

GENE ACTIVATION

GROWTH MUTANTS

In previous chapters we have mentioned several times that one of the critical steps, if not the critical step in the regulation of cellular proliferation in mammalian cells, is gene activation. It is now time to examine in some detail (a) what we mean by gene activation and (b) evidence that gene activation is a prerequisite step in the control of cell division in mammalian cells.

By gene activation we simply mean the activation (or the derepression) of a segment of the mammalian cell genome that controls the replication of DNA and the subsequent cell division. This is the same as saying that (a) in mammalian chromosomes there is a set of genes that directly and/or indirectly control cell division; (b) that these genes are not transcribed or, if transcribed, are not translated in quiescent resting cells; and (c) that they are transcribed and translated when a cell is stimulated to proliferate. The concept is naturally borrowed from microbial genetics and is simply an application to mammalian cells and cell division of the classical model of control of gene expression in bacteria enunciated several years ago by Jacob and Monod (1961). It assumes a set of repressed genes hidden somewhere in the labyrinth of the mammalian chromatin, waiting for their Theseus to derepress them.

In phages and in microorganisms, genes that control the initiation of DNA synthesis and its continuation have already been identified. The evidence has been discussed in an excellent review by Lark (1969), to which we refer the reader for specific references. Thus, the replication of T4-phage DNA is controlled by at least 20 different genes, and a number of conditional lethal mutants of *Bacillus subtilis* have been isolated which affect replication. Interestingly enough, all of the mutants contained normal amounts of deoxynucleoside triphosphates and their DNA polymerase also appeared to be thermostable, again reinforcing the evidence presented in previous chapters that the control of DNA synthesis is based on more subtle mechanisms than the concentration of DNA precursors or enzymes. Temperature-sensitive (TS) mutations resulting in a defect in either the initiation or the propagation of DNA replication at the restrictive temperature have also been described in the yeast *Saccharomyces cerevisiae* (Hartwell 1971). This topic has been discussed in a beautiful review of the genetic control of cell division in yeasts by Hartwell et al. (1974). Among the various cell cycle-specific TS mutants of *Saccharomyces cerevisiae* there is a "start"' mutant, that is, a mutant in which the thermosensitive step controls all other steps in the division cycle. After having thus acknowledged the existence of genes that control the replication of the genome in bacteria and yeasts, we must add that no such genes have been demonstrated in mammalian cells. True, Thompson and coworkers (1972) isolated a temperature-sensitive mutant of L-mouse cells that does not synthesize DNA at the nonpermissive temperature. Dulbecco and Eckhart (1970) have shown that a temperature-sensitive mutant of polyoma virus (TS-3) has a reduced ability, at the nonpermissive temperature, to induce cellular DNA synthesis in the BALB-3T3 cells. However, in both cases the mechanisms by which DNA synthesis is inhibited at the nonpermissive temperature is yet unknown. In another temperaturesensitive growth mutant of BHK cells, the defect has been identified as a mutation affecting the processing of 28S ribosomal RNA at the restrictive temperature (Toniolo et al. 1973). These results obviously suggest that the isolation of temperature-sensitive growth mutants may constitute the most direct approach for rigorous identification of gene products that regulate the transition of quiescent cells to the proliferative state. However, the isolation of the desired temperature-sensitive growth mutants of mammalian cells is a laborious procedure. Most growth mutants have fundamental lesions (such as a defect in respiration) that will cause cells to arrest at random throughout the cell cycle. To elucidate the mechanisms that control cell proliferation, one needs cell cycle-specific mutants and, presumably, mutants for very early events that occur immediately after stimulation. Some cell cycle-specific TS mutants have been isolated by Scheffler and Buttin (1973), Smith and Wigglesworth (1973), and Burstin et al. (1974), but the defect, in all cases, seems to be located late in the prereplicative phase rather than in the early stages in which we are particularly interested (see below). While waiting for these magic wands, let us recognize that although it is not unreasonable to assume that in mammalian DNA there is a set of genes that control DNA synthesis and cell division, for the moment their existence can be only inferred by analogy to microbial systems.

DEFINITION OF THE PROBLEM

There is another difference in respect to microbial cells that ought to be mentioned and that is that the size of the genome in *E. coli* is 2.8×10^9 daltons (most of which is transcribed) and in mammalian cells, 3×10^{12} daltons (5%-10% of which is transcribed). It is not surprising that in many instances regulation of gene expression in mammalian cells is somewhat more complicated than in bacteria. It is, therefore, to be expected that the regulation of gene expression in cistrons that may control DNA synthesis and cell division will depend on a number of further controls located in the cytoplasm and on the surface membrane; controls that will be the object of our discussion in later chapters. In this chapter we will be concerned n ot with the mechanisms that control gene expression in cells stimulated to proliferate, but rather with the evidence that new segments of the genome may be activated in stimulated cells. Again, we are concerned here with the initial trigger, that is, with gene activation occurring very early in the prereplicative phase of G_0 cells stimulated to proliferate. We are assuming that this is one of the critical steps, if not the critical step, that regulates the flow of G_0 cells into DNA synthesis and cell division. It goes without saying that once the cell is stimulated there may be different rounds of gene activation which may manifest themselves in the appearance of new RNA species coding for new proteins. The evidence for these alternating rounds of RNA and protein synthesis has been discussed in the previous chapter and includes the appearance of new RNA species in re-generating liver after partial hepatectomy. With gene activation defined as above, the precise question we are now posing is "What is the evidence for early gene activation in G_0 cells stimulated to proliferate?" The rest of this chapter will be devoted to a discussion of this evidence.

RNA SYNTHESIS AND ACTINOMYCIN D

The first suggestion that gene activation occurs in G_0 cells stimulated to proliferate came from the experiments of Lieberman and coworkers who showed that low doses of actinomycin D inhibited the entry of explanted rabbit kidney cells into DNA synthesis and cell division (Lieberman et al. 1963). Rabbit kidney cells are quiescent cells which ordinarily do not synthesize DNA nor divide, but can do so after a lag period of about 30 hours, when they are explanted in tissue culture under appropriate conditions. Lieberman and coworkers showed that a concentration of actinomycin D, as low as 0.01 $\mu g/ml$, almost completely inhibited the induction of DNA synthesis in explants of kidney cells. Such a concentration, per se, had no effect on the rate of RNA synthesis of quiescent cells but it did inhibit the increase in the rate of RNA synthesis that occurred when quiescent cells were stimulated to proliferate. Furthermore, such a concentration of actinomycin D did not affect the continuation of DNA synthesis in cells that had already entered the S phase. Lieberman and coworkers pointed out, with these experiments, two important pieces of evidence suggesting gene activation in stimulated G_0 cells, namely (a) that the rate of RNA synthesis increases in stimulated cells early in the prereplicative phase and (b) that the inhibitory effect of actinomycin D is not on DNA synthesis but on the flow of cells from the prereplicative phase into the S phase. These results were promptly confirmed by Lieberman's group in regenerating liver after partial hepatectomy (Fujioka et al. 1963), and since then these two phenomena have been observed and reported in a variety of situations in which quiescent cells are stimulated to proliferate, including the isoproterenol-stimulated salivary glands of mice (Baserga and Heffler 1967), phytohemagglutinin-stimulated lymphocytes (Cooper and Rubin 1965, Pogo et al. 1966), the folicacid stimulated kidney (Taylor et al. 1966, Threlfall and Taylor 1969), the estrogen-stimulated uterus (Ui and Mueller 1963, Hamilton et al. 1968), confluent monolayers of WI-38 human diploid fibroblasts stimulated to proliferate by serum (Farber et al. 1971), and erythoid cells stimulated by erythropoietin (Perretta et al. 1971, Maniatis et al. (1973).

We must refer the reader, who wishes to have further references on this topic, to a recent review by Stein and Baserga (1972). Suffice it to say here that these two phenomena (increased rate of RNA synthesis and sensitivity to low doses of actinomycin D) are generally accepted by most investigators as bona fide events occuring in the very early prereplicative phase of G_0 cells stimulated to proliferate. The problem here is not whether these two phenomena do occur as a rule, but whether they, in fact, signify gene activation. Unfortunately, neither of these two phenomena are quite convincing in this respect. The increased rate of RNA synthesis is compatible with, but does not indicate, an activation of new sites previously repressed, since an increase in RNA synthesis could also be produced by simply increasing the rate of transcription of already active genes. This is, of course, assuming that the reported increases in the rates of RNA synthesis are biochemically correct. As mentioned before, some of the reported increases are slightly extravagant because of the failure by some investigators to determine the size and specific activity of the precursor pool. But, even after the variations in pool size are taken into consideration, the figures indicate that in all models of stimulated-DNA synthesis there is an early bona fide increase in RNA synthesis. As an illustration we may take the twentyfold increase in RNA synthesis reported by Todaro et al. (1965) in

3T3 cells stimulated by a change of medium and subsequently shown, by Cunningham and Pardee (1969), to be largely due to an increase in the uptake of ^{3}H uridine by stimulated cells. However, there is a modest but real increase in RNA synthesis in 3T3 cells and, in addition, the increased synthesis of RNA in WI-38 human diploid fibroblasts stimulated by serum has been shown to be independent from changes in precursor's uptake (Farber et al. 1971). So the substantial finding that confluent monolayers of cells in culture do increase the rate of RNA synthesis when they are stimulated to proliferate remains valid, but it still does not indicate activation of new gene sites. The same criticisms apply to the findings of increased incorporation of labeled precursors into poly (a)-rich cytoplasmic RNA of phytophemagglutinin-stimulated lymphocytes (Rosenfeld et al. 1972), or WI-38 fibroblasts stimulated by nutritional changes (Novi and Baserga 1975). Here again, the increased incorporation could be explained by decreased degradation or increased speed of processing of mRNA precursors and not necessarily by the appearance in the cytoplasm of new species of mRNA.

Similarly, the effect of low doses of actinomycin D on the flow of cells from G_0 to the S phase must be taken with some reservations. In the first place, actinomycin D may have a variety of other inhibitory actions besides inhibiting DNA-dependent RNA polymerase, so that the inhibitory effect of actinomycin D could be due to other causes than the inhibition of gene expression. In some cases it is possible to overcome this objection. As mentioned in the previous chapter, in the isoproterenol-stimulated salivary gland it is possible to inhibit the stimulation of DNA synthesis without totally inhibiting macromolecular synthesis. Thus while α-amylase is resynthesized in the salivary glands of isoproterenol-treated mice, even after large doses of actinomycin D, the stimulation of DNA synthesis caused by isoproterenol is promptly suppressed by the drug. Although these findings do not tell us that actinomycin D is specifically inhibiting gene activation, it indicates at least that the action of actinomycin D has some kind of selectivity.

Another important objection to actinomycin D experiments is that the effect of actinomycin D is long lasting. For instance, in experimental animals an injection of actinomycin D may inhibit RNA synthesis for a period of 20 hours or more. In these circumstances it is somewhat difficult to decide whether the inhibition of the flow of cells from G_0 to S is due to specific inhibition of mRNA synthesis during the very early stages of the prereplicative phase or to the inhibition of, say, ribosomal RNA synthesis occurring at later times after stimulation. As mentioned in the previous chapter, there is no question that at some time during the prereplicative phase there is a stimulation of ribosomal RNA synthesis, which is particularly sensitive to low concentrations of actinomycin D (Perry and Kelley 1968).

In conclusion, although a number of investigators have devoted their time to studies of the effect of actinomycin D on induced cell proliferation and the rate of RNA synthesis after stimulation, these two phenomena, although compatible, do not give any firm indication that gene activation occurs during the very early stages of the prereplicative phase of cells stimulated to proliferate. It is, therefore, necessary to turn to other kinds of evidence to find support for the postulated gene activation.

CHROMATIN TEMPLATE ACTIVITY

Reasonable evidence supporting the concept of gene activation in stimulated cells comes from studies on chromatin template activity. Before we proceed to examine this evidence, we should spend a few words on the meaning of chromatin template activity and its relationship to actual in vivo conditions. Bonner and coworkers (1968) pioneered the finding that a preparation can be obtained from the cells of plants and animal tissues which consists of chromatin and is capable of incorporating nucleotides into RNA in an appropriate incubation mixture. The chromatin preparation can be obtained directly from cells or from purified nuclei. In either case contamination with cytoplasmic

TABLE 6.1 Protein/DNA Ratio in Various Chromatins

Tissue	Method of preparation	Protein/DNA[a]	References
Rat uterus	Directly from tissue	2.16 (0.71)	Barker and Warren (1966)
Rat liver	Directly from tissue	2.10 (0.95)	Elgin and Bonner (1970)
Rat kidney	Directly from tissue	1.65 (0.70)	Elgin and Bonner (1970)
Chicken liver	Directly from tissue	2.05 (0.88)	Elgin and Bonner (1970)
Chicken erythrocyte	Directly from tissue	1.62 (0.54)	Elgin and Bonner (1970)
Calf thymus	From purified nuclei	1.10 (0.21)	Paul and Gilmour (1968)
Chicken erythrocyte	From purified nuclei	1.30 (0.50)	Dingman and Sporn (1964)
Chicken brain	From purified nuclei	2.70 (1.90)	Dingman and Sporn (1964)
Rat liver	Directly from tissue	1.71	Tata et al. (1972)
	From purified nuclei	1.60	Tata et al. (1972)
	From "Triton" nuclei	1.36	Tata et al. (1972)
Rat uterus (ovariect.)	Directly from tissue	1.12 (0.42)	Teng and Hamilton (1968)
(hormone treated)	Directly from tissue	1.32 (0.67)	Teng and Hamilton (1968)

[a]In parenthesis is the ratio nonhistone chromosomal proteins/DNA

proteins is negligible (Dingman and Sporn 1964, Wilhelm et al.
1972, Augenlicht and Baserga 1973, Bolund and Johns 1973). The
chromatin preparation contains most of the DNA of the nucleus,
although the yields may vary from tissue to tissue and according to
the method of preparation. Generally speaking, as much as 90% of
total DNA can be recovered in the chromatin preparation. The
composition of chromatin also varies according to the method of
preparation and to the tissue used (see Table 6.1). It can be
noticed from the table that the protein/DNA ratio may vary from
1.1:1.0 to 2.7:1.0. Histones are usually in a 1:1 ratio to DNA, and
the remaining proteins are nontryptophan containing proteins
which have been called nuclear acidic proteins or better, nonhistone chromosomal proteins. Chromosomal proteins will be
discussed in more detail in the following chapter. The reader is
referred to a review by Simpson (1973) and to two recent symposia (Ciba Foundation Symposium 1975, and Cold Spring Harbor
Symposium 1974) for more general information on the structure
and function of chromatin. When a chromatin preparation is
incubated in an appropriate incubation mixture containing the
four ribonucleoside triphosphates, one of which is radioactive, as
well as Mg^{++} and Mn^{++}, the ribonucleotides are incorporated into an
acid-insoluble material which has been identified as bona fide
RNA. However, the endogenous activity of the chromatin preparation, that is, the amount of ribonucleotides incorporated by the
chromatin preparation, in the absence of an exogenous RNA
polymerase, is very small because the RNA polymerase is, in part,
lost during the isolation procedure (Bonner et al. 1968). However,
when the chromatin preparation is incubated with an exogenous
DNA-dependent RNA polymerase (usually from *E. coli* or from
Micrococcus lysodeikticus), the amount of ribonucleotides
incorporated into RNA increases markedly. Because of this
enhancement in the rate of incorporation of ribonucleotides into
RNA, chromatin template activity is usually assayed in the
presence of an exogenous RNA polymerase. The question has been
raised whether the same chromatin sites are transcribed by an
exogenous bacterial RNA polymerase that are transcribed by the
endogenous polymerase. Several investigators have reported

differences between the chromatin transcripts produced by an exogenous bacterial polymerase and those produced by a homologous polymerase (Liao and Lin 1967, Summers and Mueller 1968, Butterworth et al. 1971, Tsai and Saunders 1973) or the natural in vivo transcripts (Maryanka and Gould 1973). Differences have also been found in the K_m and V_{max} of homologous RNA polymerase and bacterial RNA polymerase for the same chromatin preparation (Keshgegian and Furth 1972). The question has been carefully examined by Reeder (1973) who, using chromatin from mouse and *Xenopus laevis*, reached the following conclusions: (a) there are sequences transcribed in the living cell that are also transcribed by *E. coli* polymerase (including the genes for ribosomal RNA); (b) there are sequences not transcribed in the cell but which *E. coli* polymerase can transcribe (spacer regions of rDNA); and (c) there are sequences not transcribed in vivo that are also inaccessible to bacterial polymerase (satellite DNA).

However, there are also data indicating that bacterial RNA polymerase does not transcribe chromatin at random. In the first place there is the very simple observation that template activity (with exogenous RNA polymerase) of chromatin from avian erythrocyte nuclei (Dingman and Sporn 1964, Bolund and Johns 1973), and trout testes undergoing spermatogenesis (Marushige and Dixon 1969) is very low. These tissues have an extremely low rate of RNA synthesis in vivo and it is comforting that the addition of an exogenous RNA polymerase does not increase the template activity of the isolated chromatin. More important, however, is the fact that chromatin from different tissues transcribe messages that by DNA/RNA hybridization techniques are indistinguishable from the tissue-specific in vivo transcripts. The evidence for at least a limited fidelity of bacterial RNA polymerase has been clearly summarized in an excellent review by MacGillivray et al. (1972), to which the reader is referred for detailed references. This evidence includes: (a) RNA transcribed from chromatin is competed out by natural RNAs isolated from the tissue from which the chromatin is prepared; (b) chromatin transcripts are tissue-specific and are not competed

out by *E. coli* RNA; and (c) results obtained with a bacterial
polymerase and the homologous polymerase are identical. Tan
and Miyagi (1970) have confirmed these conclusions with RNA
synthesized in vitro by liver chromatin and RNA synthesized in
vivo by liver. Finally, Axel et al. (1973), using duck reticulocyte
chromatin and *E. coli*RNA polymerase, synthesized an RNA
which hybridizes with DNA made from globin mRNA by reverse
transcriptase. The report of Gilmour and Paul (1973) that globin
mRNA sequences are found in RNA transcribed by *E. coli* RNA
polymerase from chromatin of mouse fetal liver but not in RNA
transcribed from brain chromatin has the same significance. Thus,
as things stand now it seems reasonable to assume that the RNA
transcribed in vitro by chromatin in the presence of exogenous
bacterial RNA polymerase is at least partially the same as that
transcribed in vivo by the same tissue, or in the words of
MacGillivray et al. (1972) "...the template properties of isolated
chromatin are related to the priming behavior of the intact nucleus
in vivo."

CHROMATIN TEMPLATE ACTIVITY
IN STIMULATED G_0 CELLS

If we, therefore, assume that chromatin template
activity is a measure of gene activity in vivo, let us see what
happens to chromatin template activity in G_0 cells stimulated to
proliferate. Barker and Warren (1966) were the first to demonstrate an increased chromatin template activity in cells stimulated
to proliferate, specifically in the estrogen-stimulated uterus, where
chromatin template activity increased as early as 2 hours after the
administration of estradiol-17β to rats. An increase in chromatin
template activity has been subsequently demonstrated in several
other populations of cells stimulated to proliferate, as listed in
Table 6.2. Aside from the references given in Table 6.2, an
increased chromatin template activity in tissues stimulated to
proliferate has been reported by: Bannai and Terayama (1967),
Mayfield and Bonner (1972), and Kostraba and Wang (1973) in
regenerating liver; Pogo et al. (1966) in stimulated lymphocytes;

TABLE 6.2 Template Activity of Chromatin in Quiescent Tissues Stimulated to Proliferate

Tissue	Stimulus	Effect[a]	References
Rat uterus (ovariect.)	Estradiol-17β	↑ (120)	Barker and Warren (1966) Teng and Hamilton (1968)
Rat prostate (castrated)	Testosterone	↑ (240)	Couch and Anderson (1973)
Oviduct immature chickens	Estradiol	↑ (120)	Cox et al. (1973)
Rat liver	Partial hepatectomy	↓ (120)	Thaler and Villee (1967)
Rat liver	Partial hepatectomy	↑ (360)	Thaler and Villee (1967)
Fibroblasts in culture	Serum	↑ (60)	Farber et al. (1972)
Mouse salivary gland	Isoproterenol	↑ (60)	Novi and Baserga (1972)
Lymphocytes	Phytohemagglutinin	↑ (240)	Hirschhorn et al. (1969)
Lens culinaris roots	Indole-3-acetic acid	↑ (90)	Teissere et al. (1973)
Rat kidney	Folic acid	↑ (60)	Brade et al. (1974)
Mammary gland	Lactation	↑ (4 days)	Barker and Ludwick (1974)

[a] ↑ increase; = no effect; ↓ decrease. The number in parenthesis is the earliest time (in minutes), in which a change was detected.

Chiu et al. (1973) in liver of rats fed the carcinogen N, N-dimethyl-*p*-(m-tolyazo) aniline; and Spelsberg et al. (1973) in chick oviducts stimulated by estrogen.

As an illustration of increased chromatin template activity in stimulated G_0 cells, let us look at confluent monolayers of WI-38 human diploid fibroblasts stimulated to proliferate by serum (Farber et al. 1971). When confluent monolayers of WI-38 cells are stimulated to proliferate, chromatin template activity promptly increases, within 1 hour after stimulation. The increase is in the order of 50%-60% and is quite reproducible. The increased chromatin template activity closely parallels the increased incorporation of uridine[^{3}H] into RNA in intact cells in culture. In these experiments chromatin was isolated from either unstimulated WI-38 cells or from stimulated cells and the chromatin template activity was determined as usual in the presence of an exogenous RNA polymerase isolated from *E. coli*. However, exactly the same results were obtained using a homologous polymerase (Farber et al. 1972). The increased template activity of chromatin isolated from stimulated cells could simply be due to a decreased ribonuclease activity or proteolytic activity of the chromatin preparation. Proper experiments were carried out and they showed that the ribonuclease activity and the proteolytic activity of chromatin preparations from cells 1 hour after stimulation were the same as in chromatin preparations obtained from unstimulated cells.

The next question to be raised is whether this increased chromatin template activity is related or not to the subsequent stimulation of DNA synthesis. The experiments by Rovera and Baserga (1973), summarized in Table 6.3, clearly indicate a correlation between extent of stimulation of cell proliferation and increased chromatin template activity in WI-38 fibroblasts. A similar correlation was found in the isoproterenol-stimulated salivary gland, where Novi and Baserga (1972) found that chromatin template activity increased between 1 and 6 hours after the administration of isoproterenol, 60%-70% above the control level of chromatin isolated from unstimulated parotid. An increase was obtained also when homogolous RNA polymerase was used instead of exogenous *E*.

TABLE 6.3   Effect of Nutritional Changes on Cell Proliferation and
Chromatin Template Activity in WI-38 Cells

Treatment	Stimulation of cell proliferation	Increase in chromatin template activity
None	—	—
Fresh medium + 0.3% serum	+	+
Conditioned medium + 10% serum	+++	+++
Fresh medium + 10% serum	++++	++++
Fresh medium + 30% serum	+++++	+++++

Adapted and modified from Rovera and Baserga (1973).

coli RNA polymerase. The template activity of liver chromatin
did not increase in mice injected with isoproterenol. The chromatin template activity of mouse parotids did not increase either
when animals were injected with pilocarpine, a sialogogue that
causes an intense salivary secretion but no stimulation of DNA
synthesis in the salivary glands. An even better experiment is af-
forded by the use of the isoproterenol analog mentioned before,
ie., 1-phenyl-2-isopropylaminoethanol. As the reader may remember, 1-phenyl-2-isopropylaminoethanol causes stimulation of DNA
synthesis in mouse parotids only when it is injected dissolved in
0.1 N HCl. When the same compound is injected dissolved in 40%
ethanol, it causes salivary gland secretion but no stimulation of
DNA synthesis. Chromatin template activity (measured 6 hours
after stimulation) was increased when mice were injected either
with isoproterenol or with 1-phenyl-2-isopropylaminoethanol dissolved in 0.1 N HC1. However, when the isoproterenol analog was
injected dissolved in 40% ethanol, there was no increase in chromatin template activity. It may be objected that the lack of increase
in chromatin template activity may be due to some toxic effect
of ethanol. However, when isoproterenol itself was injected dissolved
in 40% ethanol, chromatin template activity increased on the 6th

hour after injection. These experiments, then, clearly seem to relate
the increase in chromatin template activity during the very early
prereplicative phase of the isoproterenol-stimulated mouse parotid
to the subsequent stimulation of DNA synthesis and cell division.
Apart from the problem of exogenous RNA polymerase, objections
have been raised against the use of chromatin itself on the grounds
that chromatin preparations vary from one laboratory to another,
or (as a friend of mine put it), that chromatin is a very personal
thing, like underwear. However, the increase in chromatin template activity that follows the proliferative stimulus has also been
demonstrated with nuclear monolayers. This technique, introduced
by Tsai and Green (1973) allows the measurement of RNA synthesis
while avoiding the problem of the precursors' pool. Cells in monolayers are stripped of most of their cytoplasms with a detergent,
and the intact nuclei, still attached to the glass or plastic surface,
will synthesize RNA in situ with their own endogenous RNA polymerase. Using this technique (which substitutes nuclei to chromatin and an endogenous polymerase to a bacterial enzyme), an
increased transcriptional activity was reported within 15 minutes
after 3T6 (Mauck and Green 1973) or WI-38 cells (Bombik and
Baserga 1974) were stimulated to proliferate by serum.

It seems, therefore, reasonable to assume that the
changes in template activity detectable in isolated chromatins of
cells stimulated to proliferate are a mirror of similar changes occurring in intact nuclei and, presumably, in intact cells. This is
further supported by other experiments described below.

CHANGES IN CHROMATIN STRUCTURE

In the past few years, Ringertz and his associates published several reports indicating that structural changes can be detected in chromatin of cells stimulated to proliferate. Their studies
have been based on the microfluorometric characterization of
nucleic acids and nucleoproteins by acridine orange, a technique
that has been thoroughly discussed in its theoretical aspects by
Rigler (1966), who also suggested its relationship to measurements

of gene activity. In 1969 Rigler et al. found a marked decrease in thermal stability of deoxynucleoprotein complexes and an increase in acridine orange binding by nuclei of phytohemagglutinin-stimulated lymphocytes, 1 hour after stimulation. Similar findings were reported in chick erythrocyte nuclei activated by cell fusion (Bolund et al. 1969). For a while Ringertz' contention that dye binding could be used to measure gene activity remained *vox clamantis in deserto,* and did not seem to make much impression on the scientific community. Recently, however, evidence has been accumulating from several laboratories supporting the findings of Ringertz and his collaborators and indicating that changes in gene activity are accompanied by detectable changes in the structure of chromatin. The structural changes are of three types: (a) changes in circular dichroism spectra; (b) increased ability to bind certain intercalating dyes, such as acridine orange and ethidium bromide (Ringertz and Bolund 1969); and (c) increased ability to bind actinomycin D. The last change, first described in stimulated lymphocytes by Darzynkiewicz et al. (1969) and confirmed by other investigators (Ringertz et al. 1969, Baserga 1971), has only an ill-defined relationship to gene activity (Seligy and Lurquin 1973). Changes in circular dichroism spectra and in the binding of intercalating dyes, on the contrary, seem to give a pretty good indication of the extent of gene activity. Indeed it has been suggested that intercalating dyes, such as acridine orange and ethidium bromide, bind preferentially to localized regions of DNA that are actively involved in transcription (Sankaran and Pogell 1973). Seligy and Lurquin (1973) also found a relationship between intercalative dye binding and template activity in isolated avian chromatin.

Detectable changes in chromatin structure that could be related to gene activity and/or cell proliferation are summarized in Table 6.4, while Table 6.5 lists the reported instances of increased dye binding. From Table 6.4 one can single out instances in which structural changes of chromatin were caused by in vivo stimulation of cell proliferation, ie., PHA-stimulated lymphocytes, estrogen-stimulated chick oviduct, cell fusion, partial hepatectomy, and WI-38

TABLE 6.4 **Increased Gene Activity and Structural Changes of Chromatin**

Chromatin isolated from	Treatment	Methodology used	Change[a]		Reference
Lymphocytes	PHA-stim.	Thermal stability	Marked ↓		Rigler et al. (1969)
Chick erythrocyte nuclei	Cell fusion	Thermal stability			Bolund et al. (1969)
Chick oviduct	Estrogen	Circular dichroism	↑	Ellipticity	Spelsberg et al. (1973)
Rat liver	Fractionation	Circular dichroism	↑	Ellipticity	Polacow and Simpson (1973)
Rat liver	Isolation of euchromatin	Circular dichroism	↑	Ellipticity	Gottesfeld et al. (1974)
Rat thymus	Salt extraction	Circular dichroism	↑	Ellipticity	Wagner and Spelsberg (1971)
Gander erythrocyte	Salt extraction	Circular dichroism	↑	Ellipticity	Williams et al. (1972)
Calf liver	Salt extraction	Circular dichroism	↑	Ellipticity	Simpson and Sober (1970)
WI-38 cells	Serum-stimulation	Circular dichroism	↑	Ellipticity	Baserga et al. (1975)
Liver	Partial hepatectomy	Thermal stability	Marked ↓		Alvarez (1974)

[a] ↑Increase or ↓decrease in the parameters measured.

TABLE 6.5   Increased Dye Binding and Template Activity of Chromatin[a]

Target nuclei	In vivo stimulus or in vitro treatment	Dye[b]	References
Lymphocytes	PHA (in vivo)	↑ AO (1 hr)	Rigler et al. (1969)
Hen erythrocytes	Cell fusion	↑ AO and EB (16 hr)	Bolund et al. (1969)
Lymphocytes	PHA (in vivo)	↑ AO (1 hr)	Darzynkiewicz et al. (1969)
Kidney epithelial cells	Density-inhibition of growth	↓ AO (At confluence)	Zetterberg and Auer (1970)
3T3 cells	Serum	↑ AO (30 min)	Smets (1973)
Liver	Partial hepatectomy	↑ AO (3 hr)	Alvarez (1974)
WI-38 cells	Serum	↑ EB (15-30 min)	Nicolini and Baserga (1975)
Avian nuclei	Various degrees of template activity	↑ EB	Seligy and Lurquin (1973)
Calf thymus	Salt extraction	↑ EB	Angerer and Moudrianakis (1972)
Gander erythrocyte	Salt extraction	↑ EB	Williams et al. (1972)

[a]In all these instances a parallel variation in chromatin template activity has been concomitantly or separately demonstrated.
[b] ↑ increased or ↓ decreased binding of acridine orange (AO) or ethidium bromide (EB).

cells stimulated by serum. In lymphocytes and in WI-38 cells, the changes can be detected very early after stimulation, within the first hour. Figure 6.1 actually shows the increased ellipticity detectable in circular dichroism spectra of WI-38 chromatin at various times after stimulation by serum. A modest increase in ellipticity (in the 250-300 nm region) occurs in the first 30 minutes, but the increase is convincing only at 1 hour, and reaches a peak at 3 hours, still several hours before the onset of DNA synthesis. Other changes listed in Table 6.4 refer to treatments of chromatin (fractionation, salt extraction) that are known to cause an increase in chromatin template activity.

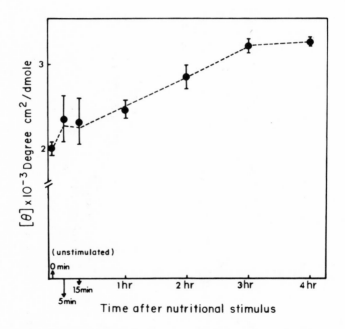

FIGURE 6.1   Changes in positive ellipticity at 272 nm of CD spectra of WI-38 chromatin at various times after quiescent confluent monolayers were stimulated to proliferate by serum. Changes in molecular ellipticity are plotted as a function of time after stimulation. Circular dichroism spectra were obtained in 0.01 M Tris, pH 8 (Nicolini and Baserga 1975).

Similar considerations can be applied to an analysis of Table 6.5, from which it is apparent that changes in chromatin template activity are parallelled by the ability of chromatin to bind intercalating dyes (an excellent review on the use of intercalating dye molecules in the study of chromatin structure can be found in Lurquin, 1974). Figure 6.2 shows the increased binding of ethidium bromide by chromatin isolated from WI-38 cells, at various times after serum stimulation. The increase is progressive and (like the increased ellipticity in circular dichroism spectra) reaches a

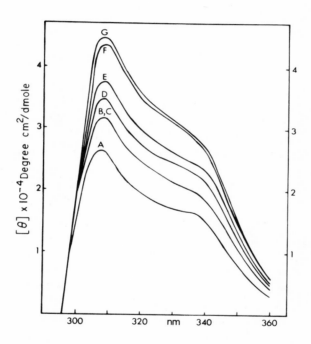

FIGURE 6.2   Circular dichroism spectra of ethidium bromide bound to chromatin from quiescent, confluent WI-38 cells (A), chromatin from WI-38 cells stimulated for 5 min. (B), chromatin from cells stimulated for 15 min. (C), chromatin from cells stimulated for 1 hr. (D), 2 hr. (E), 3 hr. (F), and 4 hr. (G). The dye/DNA-P ratio was always 0.25|±|0.01. CD spectra were obtained in 0.01 M Tris, pH 8. The ellipticity is expressed per decimole of ethidium bromide (for experimental details, see Nicolini and Baserga 1975).

maximum at 3-4 hours after stimulation, that is, 8 hours before the onset of DNA synthesis and 16-18 hours before the appearance of mitoses.

In conclusion, structural changes of chromatin (thermal stability, ellipticity in circular dichroism spectra, and increased binding of intercalating dyes) are consistently correlated to the stimulation of cell proliferation and a good case can be made for considering them a measure of gene activity (Ringertz et al. 1970). This point will be further discussed in chapter 7 where the role of nuclear proteins in determining chromatin structure and function will be taken into consideration.

APPEARANCE OF NEW RNA SPECIES

Much more substantial evidence for the activation of new genes in G_0 cells stimulated to proliferate can be gathered from the experiments of Church and McCarthy (1967), that have already been cited in the previous chapter. These authors investigated the regenerating mouse liver after partial hepatectomy and demonstrated, by DNA/RNA hybridization techniques, that 3 hours after partial hepatectomy new species of RNA appear in regenerating liver that were not present in normal liver before hepatectomy. At 6 hours after partial hepatectomy the new RNA species are essentially the same as the ones found at 3 hours but at later times, as, for instance, at 12 hours new species of RNA appear that were not present either at 3 or 6 hours, nor in normal liver. Essentially similar results were obtained by Kostraba and Wang (1973) using transcripts made in vitro by normal liver chromatin or by chromatin from a 6-hour regenerating liver. These experiments, besides giving support to the previously mentioned ping-pong mechanism of alternating rounds of RNA and protein synthesis, also seem to indicate that very early in the prereplicative phase of the regenerating liver after partial hepatectomy, there is gene activation with new sites being transcribed. These findings are of a substantial nature and the criticism often raised about DNA/RNA hybridization techinques ought to be taken with some reservations since the conclusions of Church and McCarthy (1967) and Kostraba and Wang (1973), were based on competition experiments. While it is true that the techniques used by the authors may have largely demonstrated hybridization of RNA to repetitive DNA sequences, the fact that some RNA sequences were not competed out is difficult to criticize. Church and McCarthy (1967), for instance, tried to inhibit the hybridization of RNA molecules made at 3 hours after partial hepatectomy with unlabeled RNA synthesized by normal liver. While this unlabeled RNA synthesized by normal liver effectively inhibited hybridization of labeled RNA made by normal liver, it only partially competed with RNA made by regenerating liver 3 hours after partial hepatectomy. This indicates that the nucleotide sequences of some RNA species made at 3 hours must have been considerably different from those of RNA species made by normal liver. Thus, although this is not a formal proof (as it could be obtained in bacteria) of new gene sites being transcribed, it should be considered a substantial piece of evidence that gene activation occurs at a very early stage in regenerating liver after partial hepatectomy.

An increased number of active gene sites is also suggested by the findings of Grady and Campbell (1973) with AL/N cells, a mouse cell line with a low saturation density ($7|x|10^4$ cells/cm^2). Using RNA-driven hybridization techniques, Grady and Campbell (1973) found that the same number of unique DNA sequences were expressed in subconfluent (growing) and confluent (stationary) cultures. However, a number of unique DNA sequences that were expressed in confluent cells were not expressed in growing cells and vice versa.

MECHANISMS OF INCREASED TRANSCRIPTION

The data, thus far, seem to support the hypothesis that, in cells stimulated to proliferate, there are early changes in the structure and function of chromatin that can be interpreted as an increase in transcriptional activity. Several alternatives can be

invoked to explain an increased transcriptional activity, namely:
(a) the increase is due not to an increase in RNA synthesis but to
a decreased breakdown of nuclear RNA; (b) there is an increase in
the rate of transcription, ie., a speeding up of the rate at which RNA
polymerase reads the template; (c) there is an increased number of
RNA polymerase molecules per gene site; or (d) the number of gene
sites available for transcription is increased.

Several lines of evidence indicate that heterogenous
nuclear RNA (most of which is broken down within a few minutes
after its synthesis) contains the sequences that will appear as mRNA
molecules on cytoplasmic polysomes (Firtel and Lodish 1973; see
also the lucid review by Darnell et al. 1973). It is conceivable that
certain DNA sequences are constantly transcribed, whether the
cell is resting or dividing, and that the state of the cell determines
only which transcript will be translated. According to Aloni (1972)
SV-40 DNA is symmetrically transcribed on both strands and the
unwanted sequences of each RNA strand are then degraded from
the 5' end, leading to the mature viral message. Enzymes capable
of cleaving precursor RNA into translatable message have been
described in phages (Hercules et al. 1974) and in eukaryotic cells
(Niessing and Sekeris 1973). This topic will be further discussed
in chapter 8, but for the moment we can say that this is a viable
alternative, worthy of detailed investigation.

A simple increase in the rate of transcription is unlikely,
since at least in some instances (Cox et al. 1973, Bombik and
Baserga 1974) RNA synthesis has been measured under conditions
in which RNA polymerase elongates RNA chains but does not re-
initiate, so that any difference must reflect the number of RNA
chains completed rather than rates. The third alternative is very
difficult to separate (by available methodologies) from the last
possibility, which has already been discussed above, under the sub-
heading of *New RNA Species*. We can add here that increased RNA
polymerase activity is the earliest detectable response of uterine
nuclei to stimulation by estradiol-17β (see review by O'Malley and
Means 1974); the activity of RNA polymerase II increases within
10-15 minutes, while RNA polymerase I activity increases between
30 and 60 minutes (Glasser et al. 1972). However, this could simply

be due to a modification of the enzyme or to a decrease in its rate of degradation. It would be profitable if one could apply to the estrogen-stimulated uterus the techniques developed by Chambon and coworkers (Cochet-Meilhac and Chambon 1974) for determining the number of RNA polymerase II molecules per haploid genome. This approach seems particularly promising since Cochet-Meilhac et al. (1974) have reported that the number of RNA polymerase II molecules per haploid genome in rat uterus increases from $4.7|x|10^3$ in ovariectomized rats to $1.6|x|10^4$ in mature rats.

In support of the fourth and last possibility we can mention the experiments of Hill and Baserga (1974) who found an increased number of binding sites for *E. coli* RNA polymerase in chromatin of WI-38 cells stimulated to proliferate. Some indirect evidence also comes from the observation of Abelson et al. (1974) that the rate of formation of mRNA increases in mouse fibroblasts during transition from resting to growing state.

In summary, the situation is the following. Chromatin template activity and dye binding seem to measure the extent of transcriptional activity of the genome. Whether the RNA made by an exogenous bacterial RNA polymerase is identical to the one made by the endogenous RNA polymerase is, of course, of the utmost importance. However, available data indicate that the quantitative difference detectable in chromatin template activity when an exogenous RNA poymerase is used can be reproduced with an homologous RNA polymerase or with nuclei. One is, therefore, tempted to conclude that the increase in chromatin template activity and dye binding occurring in stimulated cells is a measure of an increase in transcriptional activity of the genome. This, in addition to the experiments of Church and McCarthy (1967) on regenerating mouse liver after partial hepatectomy, constitutes the foundation for the belief that gene activation is one of the triggering events in the biochemical sequence leading from the application of the stimulus to the onset of DNA synthesis. This idea, originally formulated by Baserga in 1965, and subsequently enunciated also by Allfrey (1969) and by Lieberman (1971) receives strong support from the data gathered in this chapter.

While in future years surely more evidence will accumulate
to finally bring forth a rigorous demonstration of gene activation, one is allowed to ask now the next question, namely, what
are the mechanisms that control the activation of the genome
in cells stimulated to proliferate? The mechanism that controls
the activation of genes responsible for cellular proliferation must
be essentially similar to the mechanism that controls gene expression in mammalian cells. The problem of control of gene
activation in cells stimulated to proliferate becomes, therefore,
simply a particular instance of control of gene expression in
mammalian genes. One ought, therefore, to investigate the
mechanisms that control gene expression in mammalian cells,
with specific references to those that control cellular proliferation.
This is the subject of discussion in the next chapter.

References
Abelson, H.T., Johnson, L.F., Penman, S., and Green, H. (1974). *Cell 1:*
        162-165.
Allfrey, V.C. (1969). In *Biochemistry of Cell Division,* R. Baserga (ed.).
        Charles C. Thomas, Springfield, Ill. pp. 179-205.
Aloni, Y. (1972). *Proc. Natl. Acad. Sci. 69*:2404-2409.
Alvarez, M.R. (1974). *Exp. Cell Res. 83*: 225-203.
Angerer, L.M. and Moudrianakis, E.N. (1972). *J. Mol. Biol. 63*: 505-521.
Augenlicht, L. and Baserga, R. (1973). *Arch. Biochem. Biophys. 158*: 89-96.
Axel, R., Cedar, H., and Felsenfeld, G. (1973). *Proc. Natl. Acad. Sci. 70*:
        2029-2032.
Bannai, S. and Terayama, H. (1967). *Biochim. Biophys. Acta 142*: 410-418.
Barker, K.L. and Ludwich, T.M. (1974). *Proc. Soc. Exp. Biol. Med. 145*:
        1325-1328.
Barker, K.L. and Warren, J.C. (1966). *Proc. Natl. Acad. Sci. 56*: 1298-1302.
Baserga, R. (1965). *Cancer Res. 25*: 581-595.
Baserga, R. (1971). In *Regulation of Cell Metabolism* E. Mihich (ed.). Academic
        Press, New York, pp. 34-45.
Baserga, R., Bombik, B., and Nicolini, C. (1975). Ciba Foundation Symposium
        on The Structure and Function of Chromatin, pp. 269-278.
Baserga, R. and Heffler, S. (1967). *Exp. Cell Res. 46*: 571-580.
Bolund, L. and Johns, E.W. (1973). *Eur. J. Biochem. 40*: 591-598.
Bolund, L., Ringertz, N.R., and Harris, H. (1969). *J. Cell Sci. 4*: 71-87.

Bombik, B.M. and Baserga, R. (1974). *Proc. Natl. Acad. Sci. 71*: 2038-2042.

Bonner, J., Chalkley, G.R., Dahmus, M., Fambrough, D., Fujimura, F., Huang, R. C., Huberman, J. A., Jensen, R., Marushige, K., Ohlenbusch, H., Olivera, B. and Widholm, J. (1968). In *Methods in Enzymology*, vol. 12. Grossman, L. and Moldave, K. (eds.). Academic Press, New York, pp. 3-65.

Brade, W.P., Thomson, J.A., Chiu, J.F., and Hnilica, L.S. (1974). *Exp. Cell Res. 84*: 183-190.

Burstin, S.J., Meiss, H.K., and Basilico, C.J. (1974). *J. Cell Physiol. 84:* 397-408.

Butterworth, P.H.W., Cox, R.F., and Chesterton, C.J. (1971). *Eur. J. Biochem. 23*: 229-241.

Chiu, J., Craddock, C., Getz, S., and Hnilica, L.S. (1973). *FEBS Letters 33*: 247-250.

Church, R.B. and McCarthy, B.J. (1967). *J. Mol. Biol. 23*: 459-475.

Cochet-Meilhac, M. and Chambon, P. (1974). *Biochim. Biophys. Acta. 353*: 160-184.

Cochet-Meihac, M., Nuret, P., Courvalin, J.C., and Chambon, P. (1974). *Biochim. Biophys. Acta. 353*: 185-192.

Cold Spring Harbor Symposia on Quantitative Biology (1974). Chromosome Structure and Function, Vol. 38. Cold Spring Harbor Laboratory.

Cooper, H.L. and Rubin, A.D. (1965). *Blood 25*: 1014-1027.

Couch, R.M. and Anderson, K.M. (1973). *Biochemistry 12*: 3114-3121.

Cox, R.F., Haines, M.E. and Carey, N.H. (1973). *Eur. J. Biochem 32*: 513-524.

Cunningham, D.D. and Pardee, A.B. (1969). *Proc. Natl. Acad. Sci. 64*: 1049-1056.

Darnell, G.E., Jelinek, W.R., and Malloy, G.R. (1973). *Science 181*: 1215-1221.

Darzynkiewicz, Z., Bolund, L., and Ringertz, N.R. (1969). *Exp. Cell Res. 56*: 418-424.

Dingman, C.W. and Sporn, M.B. (1964). *J. Biol. Chem. 239*: 3483-3492.

Dulbecco, R. and Eckhart, W. (1970). *Proc. Natl. Acad. Sci. 67*: 1775-1781.

Elgin, S.C.R. and Bonner, J. (1970). *Biochemistry 9*: 4440-4447.

Farber, J., Rovera, G., and Baserga, R. (1971). *Biochem. J. 122*: 189-195.

Farber, J., Rovera, G., and Baserga, R. (1972). *Biochem. Biophys. Res. Comm. 49*: 558-562.

Firtel, R.A. and Lodish, H.F. (1973). *J. Mol. Biol. 79*: 295-314.

Fujioka, M., Koga, M., and Lieberman, I. (1963). *J. Biol. Chem. 238*: 3401-3406.

Gilmour, R. S. and Paul, J. (1973). *Proc. Natl. Acad. Sci. 70*: 3440-3442.

Glasser, S.R., Chytil, F., and Spelsberg, T.C. (1972). *Biochem. J.130*: 947-957.

Gottesfeld, J.M., Bonner, J., Radda, G.K., and Walker, I.O. (1974). *Biochemistry 13*: 2937-2945.

Grady, L.J. and Campbell, W.P. (1973). *Nature New Biol. 243*: 195-198.

Hamilton, T.H., Widnell, C.C., and Tata, J.R. (1968). *J. Biol. Chem. 243*: 408-417.

Hartwell, L.H. (1971). *J. Mol. Biol. 59*: 183-194.

Hartwell, L.H., Culotti, J., Pringle, J.R., and Reid, B.J. (1974). *Science 183*: 46-51.

Hercules, K., Schweiger, M., and Sauerbier, W. (1974). *Proc. Natl. Acad. Sci. 71*: 840-844.

Hill, B. and Baserga, R. (1974). *Biochem. J. 141*: 27-34.

Hirschhorn, R., Troll, W., Brittinger, G., and Weissmann, G. (1969). *Nature 222:* 1247-1250.

Jacob, F. and Monod, J. (1961). *J. Mol. Biol. 3*: 318-356.

Keshgegian, A.A. and Furth, J.J. (1972). *Biochem. Biophys. Res. Comm. 48*: 757-763.

Kostraba, N.C. and Wang, T.Y. (1973). *Exp. Cell Res. 80*: 291-296.

Lark, K. G. (1969). *Ann. Rev. Biochem. 38:* 569-604.

Liao, S. and Lin, A.H. (1967). *Proc. Natl. Acad. Sci. 57*: 379-386.

Lieberman, I. (1971). *In Vitro 6:* 46-55.

Lieberman, I., Abrams, R., and Ove, P. (1963). *J. Biol. Chem. 238*: 2141-2149.

Lurquin, P.F. (1974). *Chem.-Biol. Interactions 8*: 303-313.

MacGillivray, A.J., Paul, J., and Threlfall, G. (1972). *Adv. Cancer Res. 15*: 93-162.

Maniatis, G.M., Rifkind, R.A., Bank, A., and Marks, P.A. (1973). *Proc. Natl. Acad. Sci. 70*: 3189-3194.

Marushige, K. and Dixon, G.H. (1969). *Develop. Biol. 19*: 397-414.

Maryanka, D. and Gould, H. (1973). *Proc. Natl. Acad. Sci. 70:* 1161-1165.

Mauck, J.C. and Green, H. (1973). *Proc. Natl. Acad. Sci. 70*: 2819-2822.

Mayfield, J.E. and Bonner, J. (1972). *Proc. Natl. Acad. Sci. 69*: 7-10.

Nicolini, C. and Baserga, R. (1975). *Chem. Biol. Interactions 11:* 101-116.

Niessing, J. and Sekeris, C.E. (1973). *Nature New Biol. 243*: 9-12.

Novi, A.M. and Baserga, R. (1972). *J. Cell. Biol. 55*: 554-562.

Novi, A.M. and Baserga, R. (1976). *Rutgers Symposium on Fundamental Aspects of Cancer Research* (in press).

O'Malley, B.W. and Means, A.R. (1974). *Science 183*: 610-620.

Paul, J. and Gilmour, R.S. (1968). *J. Mol. Biol. 34*: 305-316.

Perretta, M., Valenzuela, A., Sage, N., and Oyanguren, C. (1971). *Arch. Biol. Med. Exp. 8*: 30-38.

Perry, R.P. and Kelley, D.E. (1968). *J. Cell Physiol. 72*: 235-246.

Pogo, A.O., Allfrey, V.G., and Mirsky, A.E. (1966). *Proc. Natl. Acad. Sci. 56*: 550-557.

Pogo, B.G.T., Allfrey, V.G., and Mirsky, A.E. (1966). *Proc. Natl. Acad. Sci. 55*: 805-812.

Polacow, I. and Simpson, R.T. (1973). *Biochem. Biophys. Res. Comm. 52*: 202-207.

Reeder, R.H. (1973). *J. Mol. Biol. 80:* 229-241.

Rigler, R. (1966). *Acta Physiol. Scand. 67 (suppl. 267)*: 3-122.

Rigler, R., Killander, D., Bolund. L., and Ringertz, N.R. (1969). *Exp. Cell Res. 55*: 215-224.

Ringertz, N.R. and Bolund, L. (1969). *Exp. Cell Res. 55*: 205-214.

Ringertz, N.R., Darzynkiewicz, A., and Bolund, L. (1969). *Exp. Cell Res. 56*: 411-417.

Ringertz, N.R., Gledhill, B.L., and Darzynkiewicz, Z. (1970). *Exp. Cell Res. 62*: 204-218.

Rosenfeld, M.G., Abrass, I.R., Mendelsohn, J., Roos, B.A., Boone, R.F., and Garren, L.D. (1972). *Proc. Natl. Acad. Sci. 69*: 2306-2311.

Rovera, G. and Baserga, R. (1973). *Exp. Cell Res. 78*: 118-126.

Sankaran, L. and Pogell, B.M. (1973). *Nature New Biol. 245*: 257-260.

Scheffler, I.E. and Buttin, G. (1973). *J. Cell. Physiol. 81*: 199-216.

Seligy, V.L. and Lurquin, P.F. (1973). *Nature New Biol. 243*: 20-21.

Simpson, R.T. (1973). *Adv. Enzymol. 38*: 41-108.

Simpson, R.T. and Sober, H.A. (1970). *Biochemistry 9*: 3103-3109.

Smets, L.A. (1973). *Exp. Cell Res. 79*: 239-243.

Smith, B.J. and Wigglesworth, N.M. (1973). *J. Cell Physiol. 82*: 339-349.

Spelsberg, T.C., Mitchell, W.M., Chytil, F., Wilson, E.M., and O'Malley, B.W. (1973). *Biochim. Biophys. Acta. 312*: 765-778.

Stein, G. and Baserga, R. (1972). *Adv. Cancer Res. 15*: 287-330.

Summers, W.P. and Mueller, G.C. (1968). *Biochim. Biophys. Acta. 169*: 316-326.

Tan, C.H. and Miyagi, M. (1970). *J. Mol. Biol. 50*: 641-653.

Tata, J.R., Hamilton, M.J., and Cole, R.D. (1972). *J. Mol. Biol. 67*: 231-246.

Taylor, D.M., Threlfall, G., and Buck, A.T. (1966). *Nature 212*: 472-474.

Teissere, M., Penon, P., and Ricard, J. (1973). *FEBS Letters 30*: 65-70.

Teng, C.S. and Hamilton, T.H. (1968). *Proc. Natl. Acad. Sci. 60*: 1410-1417.

Thaler, M.M. and Villee, C.A. (1967). *Proc. Natl. Acad. Sci. 58*: 2055-2062.

Thompson, L., Mankovitz, R., Baker, R.M., Wright, J.A., Till, J.E., Siminovitch, L., and Whitmore, G.F. (1972). *J. Cell Physiol. 78*: 431-440.

Threlfall, G. and Taylor, D.M. (1969). *Eur. J. Biochem. 8*: 591-596.

Todaro, G.J., Lazar, G.K., and Green, H. (1965). *J. Cell. Comp. Physiol. 66*: 325-333.

Toniolo, D., Meiss, H.K., and Basilico, C. (1973). *Proc. Natl. Acad. Sci. 70*: 1273-1277.

Tsai, R.L. and Green, H. (1973). *Nature New Biol. 243*: 168-169.

Tsai, M. and Saunders, G.F. (1973). *Biochem. Biophys. Res. Comm. 51*: 756-765.

Ui, H. and Mueller, G.C. (1963). *Proc. Natl. Acad. Sci. 50:* 256-260.

Wagner, T. and Spelsberg, T.C. (1971) *Biochemistry 10*: 2599.-2605.

Wilhelm, J.A., Groves, C.M., and Hnilica, L.S. (1972). *Experientia 28*: 514-516.

Williams, R.E., Lurquin, P.F., and Seligy, V.L. (1972). *Eur. J. Biochem. 29*: 426-432.

Zetterberg, A. and Auer, G. (1970). *Exp. Cell Res. 62*: 262-270.

SEVEN

CHROMOSOMAL PROTEINS

In the previous chapter it was shown that functional and structural changes of chromatin occur very early in the prereplicative phase of cells stimulated to proliferate and that these changes were in all likelihood correlated to the subsequent increase in DNA synthesis occurring at a later time. Isolated chromatin consists essentially of four components: DNA, RNA, histones, and non-histone chromosomal proteins. A change in function and structure must be due to a change in anyone of these four components. For the structure of chromatin, in general, the reader is referred to the excellent reviews by McGillivray et al. (1972) and by Simpson (1973) and to a recent Ciba Foundation Symposium on the structure and function of chromatin (1975). In this chapter we will examine the experimental evidence dealing with those changes in chromatin and its components that may be responsible for the increase in transcriptional activity. Evidence obtained in resting cells stimulated to proliferate will be given priority, but, since we have indicated in the previous chapter that gene activation in the early prereplicative phase is only a particular instance of gene regulation, we will also examine the evidence concerning the role of chromatin and/or its components in gene regulation.

ROLE OF HISTONES IN GENE EXPRESSION

For operational purpose histones are defined here as positively charged nucleoproteins, rich in arginine and lysine residues (Daly et al. 1952), and completely lacking tryptophan (Crampton et al. 1955). Nonhistone chromosomal proteins are, in this context, all other chromosomal proteins that are not histones. In rat liver chromatin, there are about $1.3|x|10^8$ histone and $2.4|x|10^7$ nonhistone polypeptide molecules per haploid genome, an average of one such molecule for every 21 and 117 base pairs of DNA, respectively (Garrard et al. 1974). Several reviews and monographs have been written on histones and other nuclear proteins, and the reader is referred for general information on these proteins to the reviews by Johns and Butler (1962), Stellwagen and Cole (1969a), De Lange and Smith (1971), MacGillivray et al., (1972), Stein and Baserga (1972), Jokela (1972), McClure and Hnilica (1972), and the monograph by Busch (1965). For the sake of clarity, we summarize in Figure 7.1 the fractionation of nuclear proteins as it is carried out, for instance, in WI-38 cells in culture. Note that chromosomal proteins constitute about 50% of the nuclear proteins, which also include ribonucleoproteins, nuclear sap (or nucleoplasmic) proteins, and proteins from the nuclear membrane. The percentages apply to WI-38 nuclei, as well as to rat liver nuclei (Jokela 1972), but vary from one type of cell to another. Since we are assuming that gene activation in cells stimulated to proliferate takes place at the level of chromatin, we shall concentrate in this chapter on chromosomal rather than on nuclear proteins, and we shall begin by looking at histones.

Histones can generally be separated into five major classes (but subfractions can be obtained), ranging in molecular weight from 11,000 to 21,000 (De Lange and Smith 1971). The five types of histones are present in each cell in roughly equimolar amounts (except for F_1 histone), and the basic aminoacids are crowded into one-half of the molecule while the other half has a

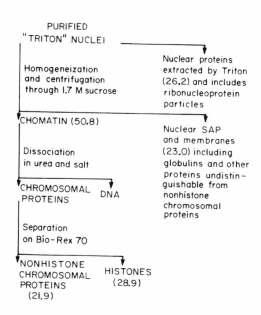

FIGURE 7.1   Diagram of fractionation of nuclear proteins from isolated nuclei of WI-38 cells in culture. Numbers in parenthesis give percentage of total nuclear proteins in each fraction.

"normal" aminoacid composition (see review by Huberman 1973). Histones are arranged in tetramers of $F2A_1$ and F3 and in oligomers of $F2A_2$ and F2B to give structure to chromatin. F_1 is a monomer and does not contribute to chromatin structure (Kornberg and Thomas 1974, Kornberg 1974). Histones have been implicated by a number of investigators as having a regulatory function on the mammalian genome (Bonner et al. 1968, Hnilica 1967, Stellwagen and Cole 1969a), not only because they are closely bound to DNA, but because in in vitro systems they inhibit DNA-dependent RNA synthesis (Allfrey et al. 1963; see also the reviews mentioned above). Although there is no question that histones are intimately involved in chromosomal structure, several important findings militate against their role as specific gene regulators, namely: (a) they are

present in similar amounts in active and inactive tissues in chromatin (Dingman and Sporn 1964); (b) they are absent in some fungi
and dinoflagellates, for instance *Neurospora crassa* (Leighton
et al. 1971); (c) there are no differences in histones between
dividing and nondividing cells within the avian erythropoietic series
series from rapidly proliferating erythroblasts to nondividing
polychromatic erythrocytes (Appels et al. 1972); and (d) they
have no tissue or species specificity (De Lange and Smith 1971).
Thus the amino acid sequence of F_{2a1} histones in two widely different tissues, such as calf thymus and pea seedlings, is essentially
the same except for two of the 102 amino acids. Histone F_3 has
135 residues, which are exactly the same in calf thymus and the
testes of the carp Letiobus bubalus, except at residue 96 where
serine in the carp replaces cysteine in calf (Hooper et al. 1973).
Specific antibodies to calf thymus F_1 histone (whose role in
mitosis has been discussed in Chapter 3) can be obtained by
immunizing rabbits with histone-RNA complexes, but other
histones do not show any organ or tissue immunospecificity
(Bustin and Stollar 1972). On this basis, the theory has been put
forward that histones are aspecific inhibitors of DNA transcription,
and that they simply act by repressing large segments of the
genome on a more or less permanent basis (Stellwagen and Cole
1969a).

This seems to be the case, also, when histones are considered in relation to cell proliferation. Synthesis of histones occurs
only during the S phase, as already discussed in chapter 2, and there
is no increase in the synthesis of histones in the prereplicative
phase of cells stimulated to proliferate. This would seem to exclude
histone synthesis as an early triggering event, but another alternative has been brought forward by a number of investigators. Histones can be acetylated, methylated, and phosphorylated (Allfrey
et al. 1964, Pogo et al. 1966, 1968, Kleinsmith et al. 1966, Patterson and Davies, 1969, and see reviews by Allfrey 1969, De Lange
and Smith, 1971, and Paik and Kim, 1971), and it has been suggested that these modifications are involved in gene regulation in general and in the regulation of cell division in particular (Allfrey

1969). Acetylation and phosphorylation of histones in the very first minutes after cells are stimulated to proliferate have been reported in phytohemagglutinin-stimulated lymphocytes (Pogo et al. 1966) and in the regenerating liver after partial hepatectomy (Pogo et al. 1968). However, several lines of evidence seem to militate against the importance of acetylation, methylation, or phosphorylation in regulating gene expression in general and cell division in particular. This evidence includes (a) histones are extensively phosphorylated and acetylated during spermiogenesis in rainbow-trout testes (Sung and Dixon 1970); but there is no RNA synthesis in sperm cells (Ozaki 1971); (b) in polytene chromosomes of Drosophila, puff formation (which is equivalent to gene activation) is dissociated from histone acetylation (Clever and Ellgaard 1970); (c) phytohemagglutinin can be divided into various fractions with different capacities. A fraction of phytohemagglutinin can stimulate DNA synthesis and cell division without causing changes in the acetylation or phosphorylation of histones and, conversely, another fraction is capable of causing these changes in histones without stimulating lymphocytes to proliferate (Monjardino and MacGillivray 1970); and (d) there is no increased acetylation of histones in the first 2 hours after WI-38 fibroblasts are stimulated to proliferate (Zardi and Baserga, unpublished data). Other evidence is discussed in the previously mentioned review by MacGillivray et al. (1972), who conclude that histone modification solely cannot explain changes in chromatin template function. In addition, returning to our specific problem of cell proliferation, there are at least two instances of quiescent cells stimulated to proliferate in which the increase in chromatin template activity has been shown to require new protein synthesis, that is, it cannot be explained purely on the basis of changes such as acetylation or phosphorylation of chromatin components. According to Rovera et al. (1971), cycloheximide inhibits the increase in chromatin template activity that occurs 1 hour after confluent monolayers of WI-38 human diploid fibroblasts are stimulated to proliferate. Interestingly enough, stimulation of chromatin template activity occurred in the presence of large doses of actinomycin D, indicating that the increase (as we shall see later), requires previous protein synthesis but not RNA synthesis. Novi and Baserga (1972) obtained similar results in the isoproterenol-stimulated salivary gland in which the increase in chromatin template activity that occurs 1 hour after the administration of isoproterenol did not occur when the animal was preinjected with another inhibitor of protein synthesis, puromycin.

Thus, the lack of tissue or species specificity and the requirement for the synthesis of new proteins seem to rule out histones as the fine regulators of gene expression necessary for the functional and structural changes in chromatin after quiescent cells are stimulated to proliferate. This should not be construed as meaning that histones are of no importance in the regulation of gene expression in general and cell proliferation in particular. In the first place they may act, as indicated above, as aspecific repressors of DNA-dependent RNA synthesis and, despite the lack of specificity their function would still be of paramount importance since they would determine if not which genes should be turned on and off, at least which genes should not be expressed on a permanent basis. Secondly, the changes caused by acetylation, methylation, and, especially, phosphorylation could be of considerable importance in determining chromatin structure, while phosphorylation itself may be associated with the transport of newly synthesized nuclear proteins into the nucleus (MacGillivray et al. 1972). It is also possible that although the specificity of gene expression may reside in nonhistone chromosomal proteins, the transcription of genes may be greatly facilitated by the appropriate phosphorylation of histones. Thus, in the lac operon system, cyclic AMP increases the phosphorylation of proteins and acts at the promoter site to facilitate initiation of transcription (Pastan and Perlman 1970). Finally, it should be mentioned that in regenerating rat liver a small but significant decrease in the amount of F_1 histone has been shown to occur within the first few hours after partial hepatectomy (Garrard and Bonner 1974).

NONHISTONE CHROMOSOMAL PROTEINS

We shall now turn our attention to the second category
of chromosomal proteins, the nonhistone chromosomal proteins.
We have defined above the nonhistone chromosomal proteins as
all nontryptophan containing proteins found in the chromosomal
structure. These proteins, after their discovery in 1946 by Mirsky
and Pollister, were largely neglected for nearly 20 years, but after
surviving frivolous claims that they did not even exist, have assumed
recently a considerable importance among students of chromosomal structure and function. Monographs and reviews on chromosomal and nuclear nonhistone proteins can be consulted by the
interested reader (Busch 1965, Stellwagen and Cole 1969a,
Baserga and Stein 1971, McClure and Hnilica 1972, MacGillivray
et al., 1972, Stein and Baserga 1972, Stein et al. 1974b, Baserga
1974). Briefly, they are usually negatively charged, are rich in
aspartic and glutamic acid residues, and contain tryptophan. They
constitute 48% of the nuclear proteins in WI-38 cells (Choe and
Rose 1974), but are fewer in amount in cells with low gene activity,
such as nucleated avian erythrocytes and sperm cells (Dingman
and Sporn 1964, Marushige and Dixon 1969). They are synthesized
in the cytoplasm (Stein and Baserga 1971) like histones (Borun
et al. 1967). They have a faster rate of turnover than histones
(Holoubek and Crocker 1968, Hancock 1969) and, at least in rat
liver, total cellular proteins (Dice and Schimke 1973). They are
located but not confined to the major groove of DNA (Simpson
1970). Some nucleoplasmic proteins are undistinguishable from
nonhistone chromosomal proteins, but others are clearly different
(Jokela 1972, Stein and Thrall 1973). Indeed, the line of demarca-
tion between nucleoplasmic and chromosomal protein is uncertain and may depend on the ionic concentration in the nucleus
that one is willing to accept as the real one (Comings and Tack
1973). At variance with histones synthesized only during the S
phase, nonhistone chromosomal proteins are synthesized throughout the cell cycle. In fact, they are synthesized throughout

the cell cycle at a constant rate, including mitosis (Stein and
Baserga 1970a, Cross 1972), although synthesis of total cellular
proteins is markedly decreased during mitosis (see chapter 3).
Also at variance with histones that can be separated into distinct electrophoretic bands, nonhistone chromosomal proteins
can only be separated into a complex electrophoretic pattern
where more than 100 bands can be easily identified (Garrard
et al. 1974). A variety of fractionation procedures have been
described, ie., on QAE — Sephadex — A25 (Richter and Sekeris
1972, Augenlicht and Baserga, 1973a), SP-Sephadex (Graziano and
Huang 1971), DEAE — cellulose (Levy et al. 1972), Sephadex
resin SEC-25 (Elgin and Bonner 1972), stepwise extraction with
urea and salt (Bekhor et al. 1974), by isoelectric focusing (Arnold
and Young 1972), Gronow and Thackrah 1973) and preparative gel
electrophoresis (Wu et al. 1972, Elgin and Hood 1973) and two-dimen
sional electrophoresis (Barrett and Gould 1973), but none of these procedures has achieved a meaningful separation in terms of function. Nonhistone chromosomal proteins are obviously a motley
crowd of polypeptides with many disparate functions besides
the property in which we are most interested here, which is to
act as gene regulators. They include RNA polymerase (which is
an acidic protein), the various DNA polymerases, proteolytic
and nucleolytic enzymes, and so on. Among specific enzymes
isolated from chromatin, we may cite poly ADP-ribose polymerase
and poly ADP-ribose glycohydrolase (Miyakawa et al. 1972), a
histone protease (Garrels et al. 1972), several protein kinases
(Kish and Kleinsmith 1974, Ruddon and Anderson 1972), the
binding protein for L-triiodothyronine (Surks et al. 1973), and
an acidic protein that specifically deacetylates histones F_{2a1}
and F_3 (Vidali et al. 1972). A list of enzymes that can be part
of chromatin may be found in the already mentioned review by
Simpson (1973). However, present day majority opinion is that
whatever else they are, nonhistone chromosomal proteins are
also regulators of gene expression. Let us now examine the evidence that supports this opinion.

NONHISTONE CHROMOSOMAL PROTEINS
AND GENE EXPRESSION

Wang (1968), should be credited for being the first in focusing the attention of investigators on nonhistone chromosomal proteins as gene regulators. He showed that the acidic proteins of chromatin restored in vitro histone-inhibited DNA-dependent RNA synthesis. The subsequent evidence supporting the role of nonhistone chromosomal proteins in the regulation of gene activity is summarized in Table 7.1 Although some of the evidence is admittedly weak, other is considerably strong, especially the experiments by Gilmour and Paul (1969, 1970). Spelsberg and Hnilica (1970), and Kostraba and Wang (1972) that have clearly indicated that nonhistone chromosomal proteins determine the organ or tissue-specificity of chromatin transcripts. In addition, it is interesting to note that at variance with histones, nonhistone chromosomal proteins are biochemically and immunologically different in various tissues and species, but especially in tissues. Thus, greater similarities were found between nonhistone chromosomal proteins of rat liver and chicken liver, than between nonhistone chromosomal proteins of chicken liver and chicken reticulocytes (Barrett and Gould 1973). There is no solid information on how these proteins interact with the genome, either directly or through histones, nor whether they act as repressors, or depressors or both. That nonhistone chromosomal proteins may act as derepressors is supported by the findings in erythroid cells of the mouse yolk sac. In these cells, 11 days after conception, only one-third of the total proteins formed are hemoglobins, but by day 13, essentially all proteins synthesized in the cell, are hemoglobins. Concomitantly, the formation of nuclear and other nonhemoglobin proteins decreases to nil between days 11 and 13 (Marks and Rifkind 1972). This would seem to indicate that for the synthesis of new messenger RNAs, erythroid cells must synthesize nuclear proteins. When the synthesis of nuclear protein ceases, the synthesis of further messenger RNA also ceases and hemoglobin synthesis continues only because hemoglobin is synthesized on a relatively stable messenger. It could be objected that repression of gene expression can also be caused by nonhistone chromosomal pro-

Table 7.1   Evidence for a Role of Nonhistone Chromosomal Proteins in the Regulation of Gene Activity

Role	References
1. NHCP restore histone-inhibited DNA-dependent RNA synthesis in vitro	Wang (1968), Spelsberg and Hnilica (1969)
2. Active tissues contain more NHCP than inactive tissues	Dingman and Sporn (1964), Marushige and Dixon (1969)
3. NHCP increase the in vitro transcription of chromatin	Wang (1970)
4. Tissue-specific nonhistone chromosomal proteins bind to DNA	Kleinsmith et al. (1970)
5. NHCP possess tissue and species specificity	
(a) By gel electrophoresis	Platz et al. (1970), Loeb and Crueuzet (1970), Elgin and Bonner (1970), MacGillivray et al. (1971), Richter and Sekeris (1972), Helmsing and Van Eupen (1973), Gonzales-Mujica and Mathias (1973)
(b) By immunological methods	Chytil and Spelsberg (1971), Zardi et al. (1974)
6. NHCP determine the organ specificity of chromatin transcription	Paul and Gilmore (1968), Spelsberg and Hnilica (1970), Kostraba and Wang (1972)

teins and that the decrease in transcriptional activity may be due to a decrease in the turnover rate of nonhistone chromosomal proteins. However, as we mentioned above, in tissues in which DNA-dependent RNA synthesis is absent or is reduced to a minimum, the amount of nonhistone chromosomal proteins is also minimal, and these combined findings would seem to suggest that the continued synthesis of nonhistone chromosomal proteins is necessary for the continuous transcriptional activity of at least some segments of the genome.

Further evidence supporting the role of nonhistone chromosomal proteins in gene expression comes from experiments on chromatin fractionation. "Active" chromatin (the chromatin fraction that contains most of the RNA synthesizing capacity) differs from "inactive" chromatin by being enriched in certain species of nonhistone chromosomal proteins (Reeck et al. 1972, Murphy et al. 1973). In some cases it has been possible to actually pinpoint, by gel electrophoresis, certain nonhistone chromosomal proteins that may be involved in specific models of gene activation. Thus, synthesis of specific nonhistone chromosomal proteins has been observed in several models of enzyme induction, as in rat liver following the injection of phenobarbital (Rudden and Rainey 1970), cortisol (Shelton and Allfrey 1970, Buck and Schauder 1970), insulin (Buck and Schauder 1970), glucagon (Enea and Allfrey 1973), and in rat kidney after the administration of aldosterone (Swaneck et al. 1970).

NONHISTONE CHROMOSOMAL PROTEINS AND CELL PROLIFERATION

Evidence that nonhistone chromosomal proteins may also be important in the regulation of cellular proliferation has come from a number of studies. Thus, Stein and Baserga (1970b) have shown that in mouse salivary glands the synthesis of nonhistone chromosomal proteins increases within 30 minutes after stimulation with isoproterenol. The increased incorporation of [3H] leucine into nonhistone chromosomal proteins was independent of changes in the pool size of precursors and reached a maximum at 12 hours after stimulation (DNA synthesis does not begin until the 20th hour after the injection of isoproterenol). Stein and

Baserga (1970b) also showed that pilocarpine, a compound that
causes secretion but no DNA synthesis, had no effect on the synthesis
of nonhistone chromosomal proteins in salivary glands of mice.
Baserga and Stein (1971) also reported the effect of 1-phenyl-2-
isoproylaminoethanol, as mentioned in the previous chapter. Just
as in the previously-mentioned experiments on the effect of this
compound on chromatin template activity, 1-phenyl-2-isopropyl-
aminoethanol caused stimulation of nonhistone chromosomal
protein synthesis only when injected, dissolved in 0.1 N HCl.
Essentially similar results have been obtained by Rovera and
Baserga (1971) with WI-38 human diploid fibroblasts stimulated
to divide by serum. This model has also been described above,
and we shall not repeat ourselves here. Suffice it to say that when
these cells are stimulated to proliferate by serum, the synthesis of
nonhistone chromosomal proteins increases as early as 30 minutes
after stimulation, remains high between 6 and 12 hours, and increases
even further at 18 hours which, in this model, is the peak of DNA
synthesis (Figure 7.2). While the synthesis of nonhistone chromosomal proteins is increased after stimulation, the synthesis of total
cellular proteins is not increased and it may be slightly decreased.
Rovera and Baserga (1973) have also shown that the increased
synthesis of nonhistone chromosomal proteins is correlated to the
subsequent stimulation of DNA synthesis. As previously mentioned,
WI-38 human diploid fibroblasts are stimulated by a change of
medium containing serum or by the addition of serum to the previously conditioned medium but not by a change to fresh medium
that contains 0.3% serum. While the synthesis of nonhistone
chromosomal proteins increased when WI-38 cells were stimulated
by fresh medium containing serum or simply by the addition of
serum to conditioned medium, there was no increase in the synthesis of nonhistone chromosomal proteins when the cells were
exposed to fresh medium containing 0.3% serum. A stimulation
of nonhistone chromosomal protein synthesis very early in the
prereplicative phase has also been reported in other situations
in which resting cells are stimulated to proliferate, as summarized
in Table 7.2 In fact, in several instances stimulation of cell proliferation or changes in growth patterns result in the appearance

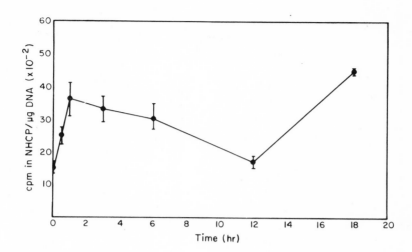

FIGURE 7.2   Synthesis of nonhistone chromosomal proteins in confluent monolayers of WI-38 fibroblasts stimulated by serum. The cells were pulse-labeled with [^{3}H]leucine for 30 min at various times after stimulation. Other experimental details are given in the original reference. Notice that under these conditions DNA synthesis in stimulated cultures does not begin until the 12th hour. (Adapted from Rovera and Baserga 1971.)

of specific classes of nonhistone chromosomal proteins (identi-fiable by gel electrophoresis) while other classes disappear. These instances are summarized in Table 7.3. There are also differences between neoplastic cells and their normal counter-parts, but these will be discussed in another chapter.

Phosphorylation of nonhistone chromosomal proteins may also play an important role in the regulation of gene expres-sion in general, and cell proliferation, in particular. Stein et al. (1974b) reviewed the evidence suggesting that gene expression may be modulated by phosphorylation of nonhistone proteins. An increased phosphorylation of nonhistone chromosomal proteins has been reported in a number of instances of stimulated cell proliferation, such as cycling HeLa cells (Karn et al. 1974), rat liver after treatment with the carcinogen N,N-dimethyl-*p*-(m-tolyazo) aniline (Chiu et al. 1973) and density-inhibited BHK

Table 7.2   Quiescent Cell Populations in which Stimulation of Cell Proliferation is Accompanied by an Early Increase in the Synthesis
of Nonhistone Chromosomal Proteins

Tissue	Stimulus	Interval (min)[a]	References
Uterus	Estrogens	480	Teng and Hamilton (1969)
Uterus (epithelium	Estradiol-17β	120	Smith et al. (1970)
Uterus (stroma)	Progesterone estrogen	240	Smith et al. (1970)
Salivary gland	Isoproterenol	30	Stein and Baserga (1970b)
Diploid fibroblasts	Serum	30	Rovera and Baserga (1971)
Mamary gland	Lactation	24 hr	Stellwagen and Cole (1969b)
Embryo fibroblasts	SV-40 infection	180	Rovera et al. (1972)
Lymphocytes	Phytohemagglutinin	60	Levy et al. (1973)
Uterus	Estrogens	60	Glasser et al. (1972)
Prostate	Androgens	24 hr	Chung and Coffey (1971)
Prostate	Androgens	240	Couch and Anderson (1973)
Liver	Partial hepatectomy	180	Pogo et al. (1968)

cells (De Morales et al. 1974), or WI-38 cells (Bombik and Baserga,
unpublished data) stimulated by serum. This topic will be further
discussed in chapter 8.

CHROMATIN RECONSTITUTION

    The evidence thus far then seems to indicate that stimu-
lation of cells to proliferate produces two important early changes:

Table 7.3   Changes in Specific Classes of nonhistone Chromosomal Proteins with Growth

Tissue	Treatment	References
Human diploid fibroblasts	Serum stimulation	Tsuboi and Baserga (1972)
Human diploid fibroblasts	Serum stimulation	Cholon and Studzinski (1974)
Immature chick oviducts	Estrogens	Spelsberg et al. (1973)
Lymphocytes	Phytohemag- glutinin	Levy et al. (1973)
Rat liver	Partial hepatectomy	Garrard and Bonner (1974)
Embryo fibroblasts	Nutritional changes	Becker and Stanners (1972)
Physarum polycephalum	Starvation	Le Stourgeon and Rusch (1971)
Physarum polycephalum	Cyst activation	Le Stourgeon et al. (1973a)
HeLa cells	Starvation	Le Stourgeon et al. (1973b)
Sea urchin	From blastomere to pluteus stage	Cognetti et al. (1972)
Chick embryo fibroblasts	Serum stimulation	Courtois et al. (1974)
Chick embryo fibroblasts	Rous sarcoma virus	Stein et al. (1974a)

(a) an increase in transcriptional activity and (b) an increase in the synthesis of nonhistone chromosomal proteins. Stein et al. (1972) correlated the two by the following experiment. Chromatin can be dissociated and reconstituted while maintaining its structure, integrity and function. Thus, Gilmour and Paul (1969) and Huang and Huang (1969) have shown that chromatin from different tis-

sues could be dissociated and, under appropriate conditions, reconstituted and still be capable of synthesizing the same RNA
synthesized by native chromatin. Similarly, O'Malley et al. (1972)
showed by immunochemical methods that reconstituted oviduct
chromatin bound a progesterone-receptor complex like intact
native oviduct chromatin. Although it may seem so at first, reconstitution of chromatin into a functional component is not
necessarily witchcraft. Tobacco mosaic virus (Butler and Klug
1971) and cucumber mosaic virus (Kaper and Geelen 1971) can
be reconstituted into functional virions by mixing in vitro their
respective RNAs and protein. Functional 30S (Traub and Nomura
1968) and 50S (Maruta et al. 1971) ribosomes can be reconstituted
by mixing ribosomal RNA with the appropriate ribosomal proteins.
Stein et al. (1972) reproduced the increase in chromatin template
activity that occurs when quiescent cells are stimulated to proliferate by reconstituting chromatin with different components. The
experiment was carried out in WI-38 human diploid fibroblasts.
Chromatin obtained from either quiescent or stimulated WI-38 cells
was dissociated in 3 M NaCl, 5 M urea, and 0.01 M Tris, and the
DNA was spun down by centrifugation. Histones and nonhistones
were separated on QAE-Sephadex and the chromatins were then reconstituted as follows. One reconstituted chromatin was made up of
HeLa cell DNA, pooled histones (pooled from unstimulated WI-38
cells and stimulated WI-38 cells), and nonhistone chromosomal
proteins from either stimulated or unstimulated cells. The chromatins were reconstituted by gradient dialysis, the template activity was measured, and the chromatin reconstituted with HeLa
cell DNA, pooled histones and nonhistones from stimulated cells
had a higher template activity than the chromatin reconstituted with
HeLa cell DNA, pooled histones, and nonhistones from unstimulated cells. The proper control (with pooled nonhistones and histones from either stimulated or unstimulated cells) showed no
difference in chromatin template activity. The results then clearly
indicated that the increase in chromatin template activity in WI-38
fibroblasts stimulated to proliferate in the very early prereplicative
phase is due to a change in nonhistone chromosomal proteins. Histones, DNA, and RNA (which spins down with DNA) do not seem

to play a significant role in this increase. Since the increase in
chromatin template activity seems also to be related to the subsequent stimulation of DNA synthesis (see above), these findings
demonstrated for the first time that nonhistone chromosomal
proteins are responsible for the initial gene activation that triggers
the sequence of biochemical events eventually leading to DNA
synthesis and cell division. Exactly similar results were obtained
in the regenerating liver by Kostraba and Wang (1973): chromatin
template activity was increased 6 hours after partial hepatectomy,
and (by chromatin reconstitution) nonhistone chromosomal proteins
are the components responsible for the increased template activity..
Comparable results have been obtained by Bolund and Johns
(1973) in crossover experiments with chromatins from calf thymus
and chick erythrocytes.

Table 7.4   **Functional and Structural Changes in Chromatin of Stimulated Cells and the Effect of Salt Extraction[a]**

Treatment	Chromatin template activity	CD at 272 nm	Percent of binding sites for ethidium bromide
Unstimulated	100	100	100
Stimulated (3 hr)	160	155	159
Unstimulated salt washed	110	68	69
Stimulated salt washed	110	73	75

[a]Quiescent confluent monolayers of WI-38 cells were used as controls (100%
values). Cells were stimulated with fresh medium plus 10% serum for 3 hr.
Salt-washed chromatins are chromatins extracted with 0.25 M NaCl. Values
are expressed in percent of values for unwashed chromatin from unstimulated cells (adapted from Baserga 1974).

SALT EXTRACTION OF CHROMATIN

Reconstitution experiments, however, are subject to criticism (Murphy et al. 1973, Choe and Carter 1974), and for this reason we attempted another approach to establish a clearer relationship between nonhistone chromosomal proteins and the changes in chromatin of cells stimulated to proliferate, specifically the progressive extraction of chromatin with increasing concentrations of NaCl (Smart and Bonner 1971). The results are summarized in Table 7.4. Extraction of both chromatins (from either stimulated or unstimulated WI-38 cells) with 0.25 M NaCl abolishes the differences in chromatin template activity (Augenlicht and Baserga 1973b), in circular dichroism spectra, and in ethidium bromide binding (Nicolini et al., 1975). Treatment with 0.25 M NaCl removes 8%-10% of the total chromosomal proteins, all of which are nonhistones (Figure 7.3), while extraction of histones begins only when the NaCl concentration reaches 0.35 M (Simpson 1973, Bolund and Johns 1973).

It should be noticed here that DNA from stimulated cells is undistinguishable by circular dichroism or ethidium bromide binding from DNA of unstimulated cells.

The results then, taken as a whole, seem to indicate a relationship between nonhistone chromosomal proteins, the changes in chromatin structure and function, the stimulation of DNA synthesis, and the burst of mitosis. As already mentioned, the initial gene activation requires previous protein synthesis and it is of particular interest to mention at this point that the initial burst of synthesis of nonhistone chromosomal proteins is insensitive to actinomycin D. This has been demonstrated in the isoproterenol-stimulated salivary glands (Stein and Baserga 1970) and in WI-38 stimulated to proliferate by a change of medium (Baserga et al. 1971), as well as in chick embryo epidermis stimulated by epidermal growth factor (Hoober and Cohen 1967). However, the insensitivity of the first round of nonhistone chromosomal protein synthesis to actinomy-

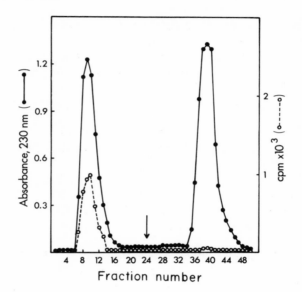

FIGURE 7.3   Fractionation of chromosomal proteins on a Bio-Rex 70 column. Exponentially growing 2RA cells were labeled with [³H] leucine. Chromatin was prepared and extracted with 0.25 M NaCl. The extracted chromatin was dissociated and the chromosomal proteins were loaded on a Bio-Rex 70 column. Absorbance values (●——●) show that chromosomal proteins distribute almost equally between nonhistones (first peak) and histones (second peak). Proteins from the 0.25 M NaCl extract, on the contrary, cochromatograph almost totally with the nonhistone peak (○ · · · ○ radioactivity).

cin D belongs to the next chapter, where we shall discuss the little we know about the cytoplasmic events that eventually lead to the activation of the genome by a nonhistone chromosomal protein.

References

Allfrey, V.G. (1969). In *Biochemistry of Cell Division,* R. Baserga (Ed.). C.C. Thomas, Springfield, pp. 179-205.
Allfrey, V.G., Faulkner, R., and Mirsky, A.E. (1964). *Proc. Natl. Acad. Sci. USA. 51:* 786-794.

Allfrey, V.G., Littau, V.C., and Mirsky, A.E. (1963). *Proc. Natl. Acad. Sci. USA 49*: 414-421.

Appels, R., Wells, J.R.E., and Williams, A.F. (1972). *J. Cell. Sci. 10*: 47-59.

Arnold, E.A. and Young, K.E. (1972). *Biochim. Biophys. Acta 257*: 482-496.

Augenlicht, L.H. and Baserga, R. (1973a). *Arch. Biochem. Biophys. 158*: 89-96.

Augenlicht, L.H. and Baserga, R. (1973b). *Transplant. Proc. 3*: 1177-1180.

Barrett, T. and Gould, H.J. (1973). *Biochim. Biophys. Acta 294*: 165-170.

Baserga, R. (1974). *Life Sciences, 15*: 1057-1071.

Baserga, R., Rovera, G., and Farber, J. (1971). *In Vitro 7*: 80-87.

Baserga, R. and Stein, G. (1971). *Fed. Proc. 30*: 1752-1759.

Becker, H. and Stanners, C.P. (1972), *J. Cell. Physiol. 80*: 51-62.

Bekhor, I., Lapeyre, J., and Kim. G. (1974). *Arch. Biochem. Biophys. 161*: 1-10.

Bolund, L. and Johns, E.W. (1973). *Eur. J. Biochem. 40*: 591-598.

Bonner, J., Dahmus, M.E., Fambrough, D., Huang, R., Marushige, K., and Tuan, D. (1968). *Science 159*: 47-55.

Borun, T.W., Scharff, M.D., and Robbins, E. (1967). *Proc. Natl. Acad. Sci. USA 58*: 1977-1983.

Buck, M.D. and Schauder, P. (1970). *Biochim. Biophys. Acta 224*: 644-646.

Busch, H. (1965). *Histones and Other Nuclear Proteins.* New York; Academic Press, *passim.*

Bustin, M. and Stollar, B.D. (1972). *J. Biol. Chem. 247*: 5716-5721.

Butler, P.J.G. and Klug, A. (1971). *Nature New Biol. 229*: 47-50.

Chiu, J., Craddock, C., Getz, S., and Hnilica, L.S. (1973). *FEBS Letters 33*: 247-250.

Choe, B.K. and Rose, N.R. (1974). *Exp. Cell Res. 83*: 261-270.

Choe, C. and Carter, D.B. (1974). *Biochem. Biophys. Res. Comm. 57*: 740-746.

Cholon, J.J. and Studzinski, G.P. (1974). *Cancer Res. 34*: 588-593.

Chung, L.W.K. and Coffey, D.S. (1971). *Biochim. Biophys. Acta. 247*: 584-596.

Chytil, F. and Spelsberg, T.C. (1971). *Nature New Biol. 233*: 215-218.

Ciba Foundation Symposium (1975). *The Structure and Function of Chromatin.* Passim.

Clever, V. and Ellgaard, E.G. (1970). *Science 169*: 373-374.

Cognetti, G., Settineri, D., and Spinelli, G. (1972). *Exp. Cell Res. 71*: 465-468.

Comings, D.E. and Tack, L.O. (1973). *Exp. Cell Res. 82*: 175-191.

Couch, R.M. and Anderson, K.M. (1973). *Biochem. Biophys. Res. Comm. 50*: 478-485.

Courtois, Y., Dastugue, B., and Kruh, J. (1974). *Exp. Cell Res. 83*: 152-158.

Crampton, C.F., Moore, S., and Stein, W.H. (1955). *J. Biol. Chem. 215*: 787-801.

Cross, M.L. (1972). *Biochem. J. 128*: 1213-1219.

Daly, M.M., Allfrey, V.G., and Mirsky, A.E. (1952). *J. Gen. Physiol. 36*: 173-179.

DeLange, R.J. and Smith, E.L. (1971). *Ann. Rev. Biochem. 40*: 279-314.

DeMorales, M.M., Blat, C., and Harel, L. (1974). *Exp. Cell Res. 86*: 111-119.

Dice, J.F. and Schimke, R.T. (1973). *Arch. Biochem. Biophys. 158*: 97-105.

Dingman, C. and Sporn, M. (1964). *J. Biol. Chem. 239*: 3483-3492.

Elgin, S.C.R. and Bonner, J. (1970). *J. Biochemistry 12*: 4440-4447.

Elgin, S.C.R. and Bonner, J. (1972). *Biochemistry 11*:772-781.

Elgin, S.C.R. and Hood, L.E. (1973). *Biochemistry 12*: 4984-4991.

Enea, V. and Allfrey, V.G. (1973). *Nature 242*: 265-267.

Garrard, W.T. and Bonner, J. (1974). *J. Biol. Chem. 249*: 5570-5579.

Garrard, W.T., Pearson, W.R., Wake, S.K. and Bonner, J. (1974). *Biochem. Biophys. Res. Comm. 58*: 50-57.

Garrels, J.I., Elgin, S.C.R., and Bonner, J. (1972). *Biochem. Biophys. Res. Comm. 46*: 545-551.

Gilmour, R.S. and Paul, J. (1969). *J. Mol. Biol. 40*: 137-139.

Gilmour, R.S. and Paul, J. (1970). *FEBS Leters 9*: 242-244.

Glasser, S.R., Chytil, F., and Spelsberg, T.C. (1972). *Biochem. J. 130*: 947-957.

Gonzalez-Mujica, F. and Mathias, A.P. (1973). *Biochem. J. 133*: 441-455.

Graziano, S.L. and Huang, R.C. (1971). *Biochemistry 10*: 4770-4777.

Gronow, M. and Thackrah, T. (1973). *Arch. Biochem. Biophys. 158*: 377-386.

Hancock, R. (1969). *J. Mol. Biol. 40*: 457-466.

Helmsing, P.J. and Van Eupen, O. (1973). *Biochim. Biophys. Acta. 308*: 154-160.

Hnilica, L.S. (1967). *Progr. Nucleic Acid Res. Mol. Biol. 7*: 25-106.

Holoubek, V. and Crocker, T.T. (1968). *Biochim. Biophys. Acta. 157*: 352-361.

Hoober, J.K. and Cohen, S. (1967). *Biochim. Biophys. Acta. 138*: 347-356.

Hooper, J.A., Smith, E.L., Sommer, K.R., and Chalkley, R. (1973). *J. Biol. Chem. 248*: 3275-3279.

Huang, R.C. and Huang, P.C. (1969). *J. Mol. Biol. 39*: 365-378.

Huberman, J.A. (1973). *Ann. Rev. Biochem. 42*: 355-378.

Johns, E.W. and Butler, J. (1962). *Biochem. J. 82*: 15-18.

Jokela, H.A. (1972). *Acta Univ. Ouluensis A. 5*: 1-65.

Kaper, J.M. and Geelen, J. L. M. C. (1971). *J. Mol. Biol. 56*: 277-294.

Karn, J., Johnson, E.M., Vidali, G., Allfrey, V.G. (1974). *J. Biol. Chem. 249*: 667-677

Kish, V.M. and Kleinsmith, L.J. (1974). *J. Biol. Chem. 249*: 750-760.

Kleinsmith, L.J., Allfrey, V.G., and Mirsky, A.E. (1966). *Science 154*: 780-781.

Kleinsmith, L.J., Heidema, J., and Carroll, A. (1970). *Nature 226*: 1025-1026.

Kornberg, R.D. (1974). *Science 184*: 868-871.

Kornberg, R.D. and Thomas, J.D. (1974). *Science 184*: 865-868.

Kostraba, N.C. and Wang, T.Y. (1972). *Biochim. Biophys. Acta 262:* 169-180.

Kostraba, N.C. and Wang, T.Y. (1973). *Exp. Cell Res. 80*: 291-296.

Leighton, J.T., Dill, B.C., Stock. J.J. and Phillips, C. (1971). *Proc. Natl. Acad. Sci. USA 68*: 677-680.

Le Stourgeon, W.M. and Rusch, H.P. (1971). *Science 174*: 1233-1236.

Le Stourgeon, W.M., Nations, C., and Rusch, H.P. (1973a). *Arch. Biochem. Biophys. 159*: 861-872.

Le Stourgeon, W.M., Wray, W., and Rusch, H.P. (1973b). *Exp. Cell Res. 79*: 487-492.

Levy, R., Levy, S., Rosenberg, S.A., and Simpson, R.T. (1973). *Biochemistry 12*: 224-228.

Levy, S., Simpson, R.T., and Sober, H.A. (1972). *Biochemistry 11*: 1547-1554.

Loeb, J.E. and Creuzet, C. (1970). *Bull. Soc. Chim. Biol. 52* : 1007-1020.

McClure, M.E. and Hnilica, L.S. (1972). *Sub-Cell Biochem. 1*: 311-332.

MacGillivray, A.J., Carroll, S., and Paul, J. (1971). *FEBS Letters 13*: 204-208.

MacGillivray, A.J., Paul, J., and Threlfall, G. (1972). *Adv. Cancer Res. 15*: 93-162.

McClure, M.E. and Hnilica, L.S. (1972). *Sub-Cell Biochem. 1*: 311-332.

Marushige, K. and Dixon, G.H. (1969). *Develop. Biol. 19*: 397-414.

Maruta, H., Tsuchiya, T., and Mizuno, D. (1971). *J. Mol. Biol. 61*: 123-134.

Mirsky, A.E. and Pollister, A.W. (1946). *J. Gen. Physiol. 30*: 117-147.

Miyakawa, N., Veda, K., and Hayahishi, O. (1972). *Biochem. Biophys. Res. Comm. 49*: 239-245.

Monjardino, J.P.P.V. and MacGillivray, A.J. (1970). *Exp. Cell Res. 60*: 1-15.

Murphy, E.C., Jr., Hall, S.H., Shepherd, J.H., and Weiser, R.S. (1973). *Biochemistry 12*: 3843-3853.

Nicolini, C., Ng, S., and Baserga, R. (1975). *Proc. Natl. Acad. Sci., 72*: 2361-2365.

Novi, A.M., and Baserga, R. (1972). *J. Cell Biol. 55*: 554-562.

O'Malley, B.W., Spelsberg, T.C., Schrader, W.T., Chytil, F., and Steggles, A.W. (1972). *Nature (London) 235*: 141-144.

Ozaki, H. (1971). *Develop. Biol. 26*: 209-219.

Paik, W.K. and Kim, S. (1971). *Science 174*: 114-119.

Pastan, I. and Perlman, R. (1970). *Science 169*: 339-344.

Patterson, B.D. and Davies, D.D. (1969). *Biochem. Biophys. Res. Comm. 34*: 791-794.

Paul, J. and Gilmour, R.S. (1968). *J. Mol. Biol. 34*: 305-316.

Platz, R.D., Kish, V.M., and Kleinsmith, L.J. (1970). *FEBS Letters 12*:38-40.

Pogo, B.G.T., Allfrey, V.G., and Mirsky, A.E. (1966). *Proc. Natl. Acad. Sci. USA 55*: 805-812.

Pogo, B.G.T., Pogo, A.O., Allfrey, V.G., and Mirsky, A.E. (1968). *Proc. Natl. Acad. Sci. USA 59*: 1337-1344.

Reeck, G.R., Simpson, R.T., and Sober, H.A. (1972). *Proc. Natl. Acad. Sci. USA 69*: 2317-2321.

Richter, K.H. and Sekeris, C.E. (1972). *Arch. Biochem. Biophys. 148*: 44-53.

Rovera, G. and Baserga, R. (1971). *J. Cell. Physiol. 77*: 201-211.

Rovera, G. and Baserga, R. (1973). *Exp. Cell Res. 78*: 118-126.

Rovera, G., Defendi, V., and Baserga, R. (1972). *Nature New Biol. 237*: 240-241.

Rovera, G., Farber, J., and Baserga, R. (1971). *Proc. Natl. Acad. Sci. USA 68*: 1725-1729.

Ruddon, R.W. and Anderson, S.L. (1972). *Biochem. Biophys. Res. Comm. 46*: 1499-1508.

Ruddon, R.W. and Rainey, C. (1970). *Biochem. Biophys. Res. Comm. 40*: 152-160.

Shelton, K. and Allfrey, V.G. (1970). *Nature (London) 288*: 132-134.

Simpson, R.T. (1970). *Biochemistry 9*: 4814-4819.

Simpson, R.T. (1973). *Adv. Enzymol. 38*: 41-108.

Smart, J.E. and Bonner, J. (1971). *J. Mol. Biol. 58*: 661-674.

Smith, J.A., Martin, L., King, R.J.B., and Vertes, M. (1970). *Biochem. J. 119*: 773-784.

Spelsberg. T.C. and Hnilica, L. (1969). *Biochim. biophys. Acta 195*: 63-75.

Spelsberg, T.C. and Hnilica, L. (1970). *Biochem. J. 120*: 435-437.

Stein, G. and Baserga, R. (1970a). *Biochem. Biophys. Res. Comm. 41*: 715-722.

Stein, G. and Baserga, R. (1970b). *J. Biol. Chem. 245*: 6097-6105.

Stein G. and Baserga, R. (1971). *Biochem. Biophys. Res. Comm. 44*: 218-233.

Stein, G. and Baserga, R. (1972). *Adv. Cancer Res. 15*: 287-330.

Stein, G., Chaudhuri, S., and Baserga, R. (1972). *J. Biol. Chem. 247*: 3918-3922.

Stein, G.S., Moscovici, G., Moscovici, C., and Mons, M. (1974a). *FEBS Letters 38*: 295-298.

Stein, G.S., Spelsberg, T.C., and Kleinsmith, L.J. (1974b). *Science 183*: 817-824.

Stein, G. and Thrall, C.L. (1973). *FEBS Letters 32*: 41-45.

Stellwagen, R.H. and Cole, R.D. (1969a). *Ann. Rev. Biochem. 38*: 951-990.

Stellwagen, R.H. and Cole, R.D. (1969b). *J. Biol. Chem. 244*: 4878-4887.

Sung, M.T. and Dixon, G.H. (1970). *Proc. Natl. Acad. Sci. USA 67*: 1616-1623.

Surks, M.I., Koerner, D., Dillman, W., and Oppenheimer, J.H. (1973). *J. Biol. Chem. 248*: 7066-7072.

Swaneck, G.E., Chu., L., and Edelman, I. (1970). *J. Biol. Chem. 245*: 5382-5389.

Teng, C. and Hamilton, T. (1970). *Proc. Natl. Acad. Sci. USA 63*: 465-472.

Traub, P. and Nomura, M. (1968). *Proc. Natl. Acad. Sci. USA 59*: 777-784.

Tsuboi, A. and Baserga, R. (1972). *J. Cell Physiol. 80*: 107-118.

Vidali, G., Boffa, L.C., and Allfrey, V.G. (1972). *J. Biol. Chem. 247*: 7364-7373.

Wang, T.Y. (1968). *Exp. Cell Res. 53*: 288-291.

Wang, T.Y. (1970). *Exp. Cell Res. 61*: 455-457.

Wu, F.C., Elgin, S.C.R., and Hood, L.E. (1973). *Biochemistry 12*: 2792-2797.

Zardi, L., Lin, J., Petersen, R.O., and Baserga, R. (1974). In *Control of Proliferation in Animal Cells,* B. Clarkson and R. Baserga (Eds.). Cold Spring Harbor Laboratory, pp. 729-741.

EIGHT

POST-TRANSCRIPTIONAL CONTROLS

TYPES OF POST-TRANSCRIPTIONAL CONTROLS

In the last two chapters we have seen evidence that when G_0 cells are stimulated to proliferate, there is activation of the genome (as measured by a variety of physicochemical techniques), which is accompanied by an increased synthesis of nonhistone chromosomal proteins. The evidence also indicated that early stimulation of the synthesis of nonhistone chromosomal proteins and the increase in chromatin template activity occurred even in the presence of large doses of actinomycin D. This was true for the isoproterenol-stimulated salivary glands of mice (Stein and Baserga 1970), as well as for resting WI-38 fibroblasts stimulated to proliferate by serum (Rovera et al. 1971, Baserga et al. 1971).

As already mentioned in the previous chapter, results obtained with antimetabolites, like actinomycin D and cycloheximide, must be accepted with reservation because the effects of most antimetabolites on cells are complex, often multiple, and only partially known. However, a negative result, in which a specific event occurs even in the presence of inhibitory concentrations of such antimetabolites, gives more information than a positive result, ie., when an event is inhibited by a drug. For instance, when the synthesis of a certain protein is inhibited by actinomycin D, it may be due to the effect actinomycin D has on DNA-dependent

RNA polymerase, but it may also be due to any one of several
side effects that actinomycin D produces in mammalian cells
(Sawicki and Godman 1971). However, when an event such
as the increased synthesis of nonhistone chromosomal proteins
in stimulated cells remains unaffected by large doses of actinomycin
D, it is reasonable to conclude that such an increase does not require previous DNA-dependent RNA synthesis. This conclusion
is supported by the finding that the increased synthesis of nonhistone
chromosomal proteins that occurs *later* in the prereplicative phase,
and more precisely after the increase in chromatin template activity
is inhibited by the previous administration of actinomycin D
(Baserga et al. 1971). Further support comes from the observation that 5-azacytidine, an analog incorporated into RNA, has the
same effect on the synthesis of nonhistone chromosomal proteins in stimulated WI-38 fibroblasts, ie., no effect on the early
increase and an inhibitory effect on the later increase (Tsuboi and
Baserga 1972).

If the early increase in the synthesis of nonhistone chromosomal proteins is independent of the genome, then its regulation must take place at a post-transcriptional level. However, in
this chapter we are not only concerned with the post-transcriptional regulation of the synthesis of nonhistone chromosomal
proteins, but also with their origin and the possible ways in which
they may modify chromatin structure and function. Thus, even
if it were rigorously proven what we have suggested in the previous chapter, ie., that nonhistone chromosomal proteins are responsible for changes in chromatin of stimulated cells, several
alternatives would be available to explain the origin of modifying
proteins. These alternatives are summarized in Figure 8.1, and
the rest of this chapter will be devoted to an analysis of the data
supporting the various possibilities.

MODIFICATION OF CHROMATIN-ASSOCIATED PROTEINS

Simpson (1973) has discussed at length the various enzymes associated with chromatin (see also chapter 6). The activity of
some of these enzymes, such as RNase, DNase, proteases, nucleoside

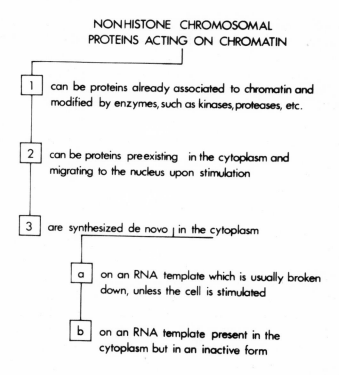

NONHISTONE CHROMOSOMAL
PROTEINS ACTING ON CHROMATIN

1 can be proteins already associated to chromatin and modified by enzymes, such as kinases, proteases, etc.

2 can be proteins preexisting in the cytoplasm and migrating to the nucleus upon stimulation

3 are synthesized de novo in the cytoplasm

a on an RNA template which is usually broken down, unless the cell is stimulated

b on an RNA template present in the cytoplasm but in an inactive form

FIGURE 8.1   Diagram of several alternatives to explain the relationship between nonhistone chromosomal proteins and chromatin structure and function in cells stimulated to proliferate.

triphosphatases, increases in aging WI-38 cells (Srivastava 1973), that is, in cells whose proliferative capacity steadily decreases. Perhaps more important is the role played by nuclear protein kinases which phosphorylate nonhistone chromosomal proteins. As many as 12 distinct protein kinase activities have been demonstrated in beef liver chromatin (Kish and Kleinsmith 1974). Some are inhibited and some are stimulated by cyclic AMP. An increase in chromatin-associated protein phosphokinase activity has been found in the isoproterenol-stimulated salivary glands of rats (Ishida and Ahmed 1974) and in the folic-acid stimulated kidney (Brade et al. 1974). In both instances, the increase occurs very early in the prereplicative phase, almost concomitant with the increase in chromatin template activity. A direct increase in the phosphorylation of nonhistone chromosomal proteins has been demonstrated in the early prereplicative phase of density-inhibited $BHK_{21}C_{13}$ cells stimulated to proliferate by a change of medium (de Morales et al. 1974) as well as in confluent WI-38 cells stimulated by serum (Bombik and Baserga, unpublished data). Although the results are fragmentary, it is possible that protein kinases and phosphorylation of nonhistone chromosomal proteins may be found to have a major role in the regulation of cell proliferation, especially in view of their importance in the regulation of gene expression in general, as already mentioned in the previous chapter.

Acetylation and deacetylation of nuclear proteins have also been proposed as a regulatory mechanism of cell proliferation. Histone acetylation has already been discussed in chapter 7, and we shall limit ourselves here to consider acetylation of nonhistone proteins. Increased acetylation of nonhistone chromosomal proteins has been reported in ovaries of rats injected with gonadotropin (Jungmann and Schweppe 1972). However, Zardi and Baserga (unpublished data) have studied confluent monolayers of WI-38 cells stimulated by serum and their conclusions, which differed, were: (a) acetate incorporation into nonhistone chromosomal proteins was modestly decreased in the first 2 hours after stimulation; (b) acetate uptake into the acid-soluble fraction of the cell was increased in the first 2 hours, and the same as in controls at later times; and (c) deacetylation of nonhistone chromosomal proteins was increased in the first few hours after stimulation. Again, the function of acetylation of nuclear proteins in cell proliferation is not clear but cannot be neglected. Like phosphorylation, its precise role will be determined only by future studies.

The same comment might apply to another chromatin-associated enzyme activity, that is, proteolytic activity. Weisenthal and Ruddon (1973) reported that the nuclei of unstimulated lymphocytes have a much higher proteolytic activity than the nuclei of stimulated lymphocytes and that certain nonhistone proteins extractable with low concentrations of salt were more sensitive to proteolytic digestion than other chromatin-associated proteins. Since proteases are known to be capable, under certain circumstances, to induce cell proliferation the possibility that they may act at the level of chromatin is attractive. Indeed, Darzynkiewicz and co-workers have found that protease inhibitors suppress the re-activation of chick erythrocyte nuclei in fused heterokaryons (Darzynkiewicz et al. 1974) as well as RNA synthesis in PHA-stimulated lymphocytes (Darzynkiewicz and Arnason 1974). Un-fortunately, protease inhibitors do not stop cells in G_1 but, on the contrary, seem to exert an effect on cells that is not cell cycle specific (Schnebli and Haemmerli 1974).

In summary, the evidence that the nonhistone chromosomal proteins responsible for the chromatin changes are modified in situ is tantalizing, but still uncertain. Other alternatives are still open.

MIGRATION TO THE NUCLEUS OF
PREEXISTING CYTOPLASMIC PROTEINS

This possibility has a precedent in the well-known fact that steroid receptors are located in the cytoplasm of target organs and migrate to the nucleus only after they interact with the specific hormone (for references see chapter 12). In this sense, one could say that at least in the case of estrogen-stimulated cell prolifera-tion the evidence already supports the migration of preexisting pro-tein from the cytoplasm to an acceptor site on chromatin. The ques-tion, here, is whether the same mechanism can be applied to other situations in which quiescent cells are stimulated to proliferate.

The demonstration by Stein and Baserga (1971) that nonhistone chromosomal proteins, at least in HeLa cells, are synthesized in the cytoplasm from which they migrate to the nucleus is compatible with the theory that the regulatory non-histone chromosomal proteins migrate from the cytoplasm to the nucleus. However, there is more compelling evidence that pro-teins responsible for gene activation, in general, specifically for gene activation related to cellular proliferation, migrate to the nu-

cleus from the cytoplasm. Some support comes from transplantation experiments in amoeba in which nuclei in different stages of
the cell cycle were transplanted into cells in S phase and DNA
synthesis was monitored by autoradiography (Prescott and Goldstein 1967). For instance, nuclei transplanted from G_2 cells into
S cells were stimulated to synthesize DNA, indicating that cytoplasmic signals in S phase cells could induce DNA synthesis in
quiescent nuclei. The experiments with amoeba leave something
to be desired because of a very high autoradiographic background,
but other experiments by Graham (1966), in which accessory
sperm nuclei were transplanted into fertilized eggs of *Xenopus
laevis,* clearly indicated that nuclei can be induced to synthesize
DNA by cytoplasmic signals. Similar results have been obtained
by cell fusion. Harris and his coworkers (Harris 1967, 1968) carried
out an extensive series of investigations on the fusion of various
types of cells, especially on the fusion of hen erythrocytes with
HeLa cells. Hen erythrocytes, although nucleated, are dead-end
cells in which no DNA synthesis or cell division occurs and where
RNA synthesis is suppressed (see also previous chapters). When
hen erythrocytes are fused with HeLa cells, the hen nuclei (but
not the cytoplasm) are incorporated into the hybrid cell, called
a *heterokaryon.* After a lag period of several hours, the hen
erythrocyte nucleus is activated, begins to synthesize RNA, and
eventually synthesizes DNA. As such, cell fusion is simply another
way by which quiescent nuclei can be stimulated to synthesize
DNA. Harris and his coworkers have shown that the stimulation
of hen erythrocyte nuclei in heterokaryons depends on the migration, into hen erythrocyte nuclei, of proteins from HeLa cell cytoplasms. Harris and his coworkers used radioactive-labeled proteins,
but an even better demonstration was recently given by Ringertz
et al. (1971) who showed, by immunological techniques, that
human nuclear proteins could be detected in chick erythrocyte
nuclei reactivated by fusion with HeLa cells (which are of human
origin). This indicated that nuclear proteins from HeLa cells could
migrate through the cytoplasm of the heterokaryon to the chick
nucleus. The migration of nucleoplasmic antigens was correlated
with the ability of the fused chick erythrocyte nucleus to synthesize

RNA (Carlsson et al. 1973), and a similar movement of cytoplasmic proteins from *Xenopus laevis* egg cells was noted when brain nuclei were injected (and thus activated) into eggs (Merriam 1969).

In another series of experiments from Ringertz' laboratory, it was reported that chick erythrocyte nuclei reactivated by fusion with HeLa cells, took up very rapidly preexisting and newly synthesized proteins from the cytoplasm of HeLa cells (Appels et al. 1974a). In the first few minutes after fusion, preexisting HeLa proteins were predominantly migrating to the chick nucleus but, after several minutes, proteins synthesized after fusion made their appearance in the reactivating nucleus. The great majority of these proteins were identified as nonhistone proteins (Appels et al., 1974b).

A massive migration of proteins into the cell nucleus was also demonstrated in trypsinized explants of mouse kidney. DNA synthesis in these explants begins after 24 hours, but during the prereplicative phase the amount of nuclear proteins increases three-to fourfold (Auer and Zetterberg 1972). A 50% increase in the amount of nuclear proteins has also been reported in lymphocytes stimulated by concanavalin A (Johnson et al. 1974), and in confluent monolayers of WI-38 cells trypsinized and replated at a lower density (Maizel et al. 1975). Finally, Choe and Rose (1973) and Allfrey et al. (1974) found a migration, into the nuclei of cells stimulated to proliferate, of nonhistone proteins capable of binding to DNA.

In all of these cases, the evidence supported the theory that preexisting cytoplasmic proteins migrated into the nucleus upon stimulation. However, the length of the prereplicative phase seems to be a major factor in these findings. Thus, in all cases in which massive migration of preexisting proteins into nuclei has been reported, the length of the prereplicative phase was rather long, from a minimum of 18 hours in trypsinized WI-38 cells to 24 hours or more in lymphocytes, chick nuclei, and so on.

Interestingly enough we have never been able to demonstrate appreciable transfer of prelabeled proteins from the cytoplasm to the nucleus in confluent monolayers of WI-38 cells stimulated by serum, in which the interval between the stimulus and the onset of DNA synthesis is 12 hours. Perhaps one could speculate that in cells with a long prereplicative phase, nuclear migration of preexisting cytoplasmic proteins is a necessary prerequisite for the reactivation of chromatin, reactivation which is then sustained by newly synthesized nonhistone proteins. The latter ones would be sufficient in the case of stimulated cells with a shorter prereplicative phase. This theory has as a corollary that cells with a long prereplicative phase have lost from the nucleus certain nonhistone proteins still present in resting cells with a short prereplicative phase. Indeed, when resting WI-38 cells are trypsinized (a procedure that lengthens the prereplicative phase in comparison to serum stimulation), their nuclei lose about 40% of the proteins, which are restored to the nucleus at later hours (Maizel et al. 1975). This interpretation could reconcile the alternative of nuclear migration of preexisting cytoplasmic proteins with the alternative of de novo synthesis of nonhistone proteins, to be discussed below.

DE NOVO SYNTHESIS OF NONHISTONE PROTEINS

Evidence that changes in chromatin structure and function in cells stimulated to proliferate is regulated by de novo synthesized nonhistone proteins is based essentially on two types of findings: (a) the increased synthesis of nonhistone chromosomal proteins reported in several situations in which resting cells are stimulated to proliferate; and (b) the inhibitory effect of cycloheximide on the increased chromatin template activity observed in stimulated WI-38 cells (Rovera et al. 1971). Both points have been discussed in the previous chapter, and both points only provide, at best, circumstantial evidence. However, it is a possibility that must be taken into consideration, together with other alternatives, until further experimentation clarifies the problem.

If new nonhistone proteins are synthesized upon stimulation, their synthesis must be regulated at the post-transcriptional level, as discussed at the beginning of this chapter. This presupposes an RNA template that is not available for translation, unless the cell is stimulated. However, the mechanism through which a preexisting mRNA is activated (or not broken down) is obscure. It should be noted, though, that precedents for possible mechanisms are already available in the literature.

The first mechanism is a purely translational control, ie., a preexisting RNA template inactive in the cytoplasm of quiescent G_0 cells. The preexisting RNA template is then somehow activated by the stimulus to proliferate and is translated into a nonhistone chromosomal protein, which then migrates to the nucleus where it activates the genome. A second possibility is that envisaged by Tomkins and his collaborators (Tomkins et al. 1972) for the induction of tyrosine aminotransferase in cultured hepatoma cells in which a second messenger RNA controls the translation of the RNA template for tyrosine aminotransferase. A third possibility is that described by Aloni (1972) for gene expression in SV-40 virus in which both standards of the genome are transcribed but only those RNA sequences to be translated are conserved, while the others are broken down before they leave the nucleus. Finally, it may be possible that the nonhistone chromosomal protein in question is always being synthesized, even in the cytoplasm of quiescent cells, but is broken down or somehow cannot reach the nucleus. The remainder of this chapter will be devoted to an examination of available data in support of the first two of these possibilities. The third one has been discussed in chapters 6 and 7, and the last one has yet to gain recognition by its first piece of supporting evidence.

INACTIVE mRNA TEMPLATES

A number of enzymes whose synthesis can be stimulated without previous DNA-directed RNA synthesis have been described in the literature. Enzyme systems that are regulated at a post-transcriptional level have been discussed by Harris (1968) in his book, *Nucleus and Cytoplasm,* and another well-known example is the one described in detail by Tomkins and coworkers (1972), ie., the induction, by cortisol, of tyrosine aminotransferase in hepatoma cells in culture. These authors have also reviewed several other systems, to which we may add catalase synthesis in liver regulated by inhibiting and activating factors that bind specifically to polyribosomes synthesizing catalase (Uenoyama and Ono 1973). All of these systems presume a preexisting mRNA which is present in the cytoplasm in an inactive or masked form until activated by a given stimulus. Such a masked mRNA specific for microtubular proteins has been described in the fertilized sea urchin egg by Raff et al. (1972), and its anatomy has been analyzed in detail in L-mouse cells by Schochetman and Perry (1972). These authors have shown that mRNA on polyribosomes of L-mouse cells can be shifted to an inactive form (in the monomer or in a not-better identified ribonucleoprotein particle) by a temperature shift. A temperature shift to 42° causes a breakdown of polyribosomes without a breakdown of mRNA, which is simply shifted to an inactive form. When the heat-shocked cells are incubated again at the permissive temperature (37°), the polysomes reaggregate and the mRNA again shifts from the monomer to the polysome fraction. This return to an active form occurs in the presence of actinomycin D, indicating that the reconstitution of polyribosomes and the shift of mRNA from a monomer to a polysome fraction is independent of DNA-directed RNA synthesis. A similar situation has been described in the unfertilized sea urchin egg, which contains preexisting preadenylated genetic messages, predominantly located in the postpolysomal fraction. Fertilization causes a rapid transfer of the preexisting messages from the postpolysomal to the polysomal fraction, without de novo RNA synthesis (Slater et al. 1973) and, at the most, with polyadenylation of preexisting messages (Wilt 1973). It has been hypothesized that a masked mRNA similar to the one observed in heat-shocked cells and in sea urchin eggs may also be present in normal eukaryotic cells (at least for certain specific situations) and that its activation may lead to the synthesis of new proteins without previous RNA synthesis.

If this were also true for resting and proliferating cells, then in cells stimulated to proliferate, there ought to be a reaggregation of monomers into polysomes. This has, in fact, been described in regenerating liver by Zweig and Grisham (1971) and by Webb et al. (1966) and in phytohemagglutinin-stimulated lymphocytes by Kay et al. (1971). Unfortunately, in both instances the reaggregation of ribosomes into polysomes is a late event in the pre-replicative phase, occurring 10 hours or more after stimulation. More significant are the experiments of Cohen and Stastny (1968) with epidermal growth factor, which caused formation of polysomes with a corresponding decrease in the fraction of monosomes in cultures chick embryo epidermis within 1 hour after stimulation. The shift to polysomes occurred even in the presence of cycloheximide or actinomycin D, again indicating that reaggregation of polysomes was independent of DNA-directed RNA synthesis. Similar results were reported by Hogan and Korner (1968) who showed reaggregation of polysomes when Landschutz ascites cells were transferred from the peritoneal cavity of mice to Eagle's medium or when amino acids were injected into the peritoneal cavity. The reaggregation of polysomes under such conditions occurred as early as 30 minutes after the cells were stimulated and, again, was insensitive to actinomycin D.

However, the most intriguing experiments in this regard are those of Soeiro and Amos (1966), who studied protein synthesis in primary cultures of chick embryo cells deprived of serum. When chick embryo cells are deprived of serum, growth ceases and protein synthesis decreases. Soeiro and Amos (1966) showed that after serum deprivation the polysomes of chick embryo cells did not break down but ceased functioning (as measured by amino acid incorporation in vivo). When serum was added, protein synthesis promptly increased and so did the activity of polysomes, the increase being insensitive to actinomycin D. Soeiro and Amos (1966) also found that the inactive polysomes were insensitive to in vitro stimulation by poly. U. This lack of stimulation by poly. U suggested that serum-deprived cells contain an inhibitor (or the absence of an activator), the function of which is altered by serum itself. Becker et al. (1971) and

Whelly and Barker (1974) went one step further and showed an increase in the number of active ribosomes (ribosomes engaged in protein synthesis) in stimulated G_0 cells, the former in cultured hamster embryo cells, the latter in the estrogen-stimulated uterus.

Summarizing the situation up to this point, we may say that the evidence for an initial post-transcriptional step in the regulation of cell proliferation rests on the findings that gene activation occurs in the presence of large doses of actinomycin D and that cytoplasmic signals may alter gene function. A possible mechanism for cytoplasmic control could be the activation of a masked mRNA, with consequent reaggregation of polysomes and synthesis of the protein(s) required for gene activation. Unfortunately, one of the steps most difficult to explain is how a specific masked mRNA can be activated among the presumably numerous masked mRNAs that exist in a quiescent cell. However, it has been reported in bacteria that certain initiation factors for protein synthesis can be highly specific. For instance, there are initiation factors that allow the translation of a phage mRNA but not the translation of the mRNA of the host *E. coli* cells (Lee-Huang and Ochoa 1971). It is possible that specific initiation factors may be activated by the stimulus to proliferate and thus activate preexisting masked mRNA-protein complexes.

LOSS OF CYTOPLASMIC PROTEINS

Another possible explanation can be found in an opposite mechanism, the loss of an inhibitor rather than the acquisition of an activator. It has been known for a long time that in several situations in which quiescent cells are stimulated to proliferate, one of the very early events is a loss of cytoplasmic components, especially cytoplasmic proteins. For instance, in phytohemagglutinin-stimulated lymphocytes, Fisher and Mueller (1968) reported the loss of gamma globulins, while partial hepatectomy causes an increased secretion of albumin from hepatocytes (Majumdar et al. 1967). In fact, according to Sudweeks and Hill (1967), it is possible to induce DNA synthesis in hepatocytes by plasmapheresis, a procedure that causes a marked secretion of albumin and other plasma proteins from hepatocytes into the blood stream. Similarly, there is no question that in the isoproterenol-stimulated salivary gland there is a loss of cytoplasmic proteins, since the glands are stimulated to secrete copiously (Byrt 1966), and Wiebel and Baserga (1969) have shown that in WI-38 human diploid fibroblasts stimulated to proliferate by serum, there is a substantial loss of free amino acids from the cytoplasmic pool. The disappearance of an inhibitor upon stimulation is suggested by the experiments of Whelly and Barker (1974) who found, in the estrogen-stimulated uterus, that the rate of peptide elongation increased before the number of active ribosomes would increase.

It is also interesting to note that transformed cells in culture are often "leaky" and, for instance, they secrete increased amounts of lactic dehydrogenase when compared to their normal untransformed counterparts (Bissell et al. 1971). These data indicate that wnen cells are stimulated to proliferate, cytoplasmic proteins and other cytoplasmic components are often lost. It is possible that among the proteins lost by the cell immediately after the stimulus is applied may be a hypothetical inhibitor directly acting on the translation of the mRNA regulating the synthesis of a nonhistone chromosomal protein. The inhibitor does not necessarily have to be lost from the cell. It could be fixed to the cell membrane, much in the same way as certain protein synthesis initiation factors are sequestered on to the cell membrane by the diphtheria toxin (Gill et al. 1969). In this latter model the diphtheria toxin, a potent inhibitor of protein synthesis, does not by itself penetrate the cell but, instead, attaches itself to the membrane where it causes a change which, in turn, leads to the sequestration of a protein synthesis initiation factor. This alternative is particularly attractive because it would directly involve the membrane of the cell, a structure whose importance in the regulation of cell division will be discussed in the next chapter.

In conclusion it would seem that in order to explain the initial round of nonhistone chromosomal protein synthesis, one has to invoke a post-transcriptional step. Among the various alternatives,

three seem to merit more attention: (a) the enzymatic modification
of preexisting chromatin-associated proteins; (b) the migration to the
nucleus of preexisting cytoplasmic proteins; and (c) the existence of
a masked mRNA activated either by a specific activator or by loss of
a specific inhibitor. The cytoplasmic changes are, in turn, mediated
by changes, either structural or functional, in the cell membrane.

References

Allfrey, V.G., Inoue, A., Karn, J., Johnson, E.M., and Vidali, G. (1974). *Cold Spring Harbor Symposia* vol. 38. pp. 785-801.
Aloni, Y. (1972). *Proc. Natl. Acad. Sci. USA 69*: 2404-2409.
Appels, R., Bolund, L., and Ringertz, N.R. (1974b). *J. Mol. Biol. 87*: 339-355.
Appels, R., Bolund, L., Goto, S., and Ringertz, N.R. (1974a). *Exp. Cell Res. 85*: 182-190.
Auer, G. and Zetterberg, A. (1972). *Exp. Cell Res. 75*: 245-253.
Baserga, R., Rovera, G., and Farber, J. (1971). *In Vitro 7*: 80-87.
Becker, H., Stanners, C.P., and Kudlow, J.E. (1971). *J. Cell Physiol. 77*: 43-50.
Bissell, M.J., Rubin, H., and Hatie, C. (1971). *Exp. Cell Res. 68*: 404-410.
Brade, W.P., Thomson, J.A., Chiu, J.F., and Hnilica, L.S. (1974). *Exp. Cell Res. 84*: 183-190.
Byrt, P. (1966). *Nature 212*: 1212-1215.
Carlsson, S.A., Moore, G.P.M., and Ringertz, N.R. (1973). *Exp. Cell Res. 76*: 234-241.
Choe, B.K. and Rose, N.R. (1973). *Exp. Cell Res. 83*: 271-280.
Cohen, S. and Stastny, M. (1968). *Biochim. Biophys. Acta. 166*: 427-437
Darzynkiewicz, Z. and Arnason, B.G.W. (1974). *Exp. Cell Res. 85*: 95-104.
Darzynkiewicz, Z., Chelmicka-Szorc, E., and Arnason, B.G.W. (1974). *Proc. Natl. Acad. Sci. USA 71*: 644-647.
de Morales, M.M., Blat, C., and Harel, L. (1974). *Exp. Cell Res. 86*: 111-119.
Fisher, D.B. and Mueller, G.C. (1968). *Proc. Natl. Acad. Sci. USA 60*: 1396-1402.
Gill, D.M., Pappenheimer, A.M. Jr., and Baseman, J.P. (1969). *Cold Spring Harbor Symposium Quant. Biol. 34*: 595-602.
Graham, C.F. (1966). *J. Cell Sci. 1*: 363-374.
Harris, H. (1967). *J. Cell Sci. 2*: 23-32.
Harris, H. (1968). *Nucleus and Cytoplasm.* Clarendon Press, Oxford, pp. 13-14.
Hogan, B.L.M. and Korner, A. (1968). *Biochim. Biophys. Acta 169*: 129-138.

Ishida, H. and Ahmed, K. (1974). *Exp. Cell Res. 84*: 127-136.
Johnson, E.M., Karn, J., and Allfrey, V.G. (1974). *J. Biol. Chem. 249*: 4990-4999.
Jungmann, R. and Schweppe, J.S. (1972). *J. Biol. Chem. 247*: 5535-5542.
Kay, J.E., Ahern, T., and Atkins, M. (1971). *Biochim. Biophys. Acta 247*: 322-334.
Kish, V.M. and Kleinsmith, L.J. (1974). *J. Biol. Chem. 249*: 750-760.
Lee-Huang, S. and Ochoa, S. (1971). *Nature New Biol. 234*: 236-239.
Maizel, A., Nicolini, C., and Baserga., R. (1975).*J. Cell Physiol. 86*: 71-82.
Majumdar, C., Tsukada, K., and Lieberman, I. (1967). *J. Biol. Chem. 242*: 700-704.
Merriam, R.W. (1969). *J. Cell Sci. 5*: 333-349.
Prescott, D.M. and Goldstein, L. (1967). *Science 155*: 469-470.
Raff, R.A., Colot, H.V., Selvig, S.E., and Gross, P.R. (1972). *Nature 235*: 211-214.
Ringertz, N.R., Carlsson, S., Ege, T., and Bolund, L. (1971). *Proc. Natl. Acad. Sci. USA 68*: 3228-3232.
Rovera, G. and Baserga, R. (1971). *J. Cell. Physiol. 77*: 201-212.
Rovera, G., Farber, J., and Baserga, R. (1971). *Proc. Natl. Acad. Sci. USA 68*: 1725-1729.
Sawicki, S.G. and Godman, G.C. (1971). *J. Cell Biol. 50*: 746-761.
Schnebli, H.P. and Haemmerli, G. (1974). *Nature 248*: 150-151.
Schochetman, G. and Perry, R.P. (1972). *J. Mol. Biol. 63*: 577-590.
Simpson, R.T. (1973). *Adv. Enzymol. 38*: 41-108.
Slater, I., Gillespie, D., and Slater, D.W. (1973). *Proc. Natl. Acad. Sci. USA 70*: 406-411.
Soeiro, R. and Amos, H. (1966). *Science 154*: 662-665.
Srivastava, B.I.S. (1973). *Exp. Cell Res. 80*: 305-312.
Stein, G. and Baserga, R. (1970). *J. Biol. Chem. 245: 6097-6105.*
Stein, G. and Baserga, R. (1971). *Biochem. Biophys. Res. Comm. 44*: 218-223.
Sudweeks, A.D. and Hill, R.B. (1967). *J. Cell Biol. 34*: 404-406.
Tomkins, G.M., Levinson, B.B., Baxter, J.D., and Dethlefsen, L. (1972). *Nature New Biol. 239*: 9-14.
Tsuboi, A., and Baserga, R. (1972). *J. Cell Physiol. 80*: 107-118.
Uenoyama, K. and Ono, T. (1973). *J. Mol. Biol. 74*: 453-466.
Webb, T.E., Blobel, G., and Potter, V.R. (1966). *Cancer Res. 26*: 253-257.
Weisenthal, L.M. and Ruddon, R.W. (1973). *Cancer Res. 33*: 2923-2935.
Whelly, S.M. and Barker, K.L. (1974). *Biochemistry 13*: 341-346.
Wiebel, F. and Baserga, R. (1969). *J. Cell Physiol. 74*: 191-202.
Wilt, F.H. (1973). *Proc. Natl. Acad. Sci. USA 70*: 2345-2349.
Zweig, M. and Grisham, J.W. (1971). *Biochim. Biophys. Acta 246*: 70-80.

NINE

THE ROLE OF MEMBRANES

CONTACT-INHIBITION OF GROWTH

The role of cell membranes in the control of cell division in mammalian cells has been adequately reviewed (up to 1972) by Pardee (1971) and by Burger (1972), and the present discussion is essentially based on their review articles, with the addition of more recent findings.

The current interest in the relation of cell membranes to cell division and neoplasia stems primarily from the pioneer work on cell movement in vitro by Abercrombie and Ambrose (1962). These investigators noticed that untransformed normal cells in culture stopped growing when they formed a confluent monolayer on a glass (or plastic) surface. This phenomenon, which was called by Abercrombie and Ambrose (1962), *contact inhibition of growth* or *density-dependent inhibition of growth,* did not occur if the confluent monolayers were refed with fresh serum. Under the same culture conditions, tumor cells did not show density-dependent inhibition of growth but rather grew to form multilayers of cells. Some of the factors that may be involved in density-dependent inhibition of growth, such as serum factors, short-range effects, and anchorage dependence of cells, have already been discussed by Stoker (1969). Ponten (1971) divides the several explanations that have been offered for contact-inhibition of growth into three categories: (a) nonspecific medium-depletion; (b) release of factors inhibiting cell division; and (c) physical contact between cells. Although favoring the third explanation, Ponten (1971) admits that the data are still too contradictory to permit any firm conclusions. Despite the mystery that still surrounds contact-inhibition of growth, the original observation of Abercrombie and Ambrose (1962), and the numerous investigations that followed eventually led to the suggestion that the molecular defect responsible for uncontrolled cell growth might reside in the cell membrane (Pardee 1964). Membrane changes in proliferating cells will therefore be the topic of this chapter, while the growth factors that may regulate cell division through membranes will be discussed in the following chapter.

While a considerable amount of work has been done on the functional and structural changes occurring on the surface membranes of cancer cells, especially virally-transformed cells, more limited information is available on the changes that take place in normal cells during the cell cycle, or when quiescent G_0 cells are stimulated to proliferate by an appropriate stimulus. We will begin by reviewing briefly the changes that have been described in the surface membranes of transformed cells and we shall then examine, in more detail, functional and structural changes that have been described in the cell membrane of proliferating cells during the cell cycle.

MEMBRANE CHANGES IN NEOPLASTIC CELLS

Burger (1972) has discussed in detail the relationship, for a variety of cell lines in culture, between density-dependent inhibition of growth and agglutininability by certain plant lectins, expecially wheat germ agglutinin and concanavalin A (see also Weber 1973). Thus, cells like 3T3 mouse fibroblasts that grow to lower saturation densities, in the order of $5|x|10^4$ cells per square centimeter, are only weakly agglutinated by wheat germ agglutinin, while SV-101 cells, which are 3T3 cells transformed by SV-40

virus, grow to a saturation density of $5|x|10^5$ cells per square
centimeter, and are markedly agglutinated by plant lectins. Eckhart
et al. (1971) used a temperature-sensitive polyoma virus mutant,
which cannot maintain the transformed state in 3T3 cells at high
temperature, and the loss of the transformed state at the nonpermissive temperature was paralleled by decreased agglutinability
with either wheat germ agglutinin or concanavlin A. The wheat
germ agglutinin receptor is apparently a glycoprotein which contains glucosamine and, interestingly enough, it is also present in
normal cells with low saturation densities. However, in normal
cells the receptor is present in a masked form and can be un-
masked only when the cell surface is subjected to brief treatment
with low concentrations of a protease (Burger 1969). Several
other investigations support the concept that the receptor for
plant agglutinins is present in normal cells in a masked form. Thus,
Häyry and Defendi (1970) demonstrated that what was earlier
believed to be an SV-40 virus-specific surface antigen was actually
present in uninfected hamster cells and was exposed by treatment
with trypsin. Protease treatment of cell surfaces also exposed the
normal cell's receptor site for another agglutinin, concanavalin A
(Inbar and Sachs 1969), as well as certain glycolipids of the membrane that could easily be detected in transformed cells (Hakomori
et al. 1968). Finally, Burger (1971) has shown that the Forssman
antigen that can be induced in BHK cells during transformation, is
present also in nontransformed BHK cells and again can be exposed by previous treatment with a protease. Indeed, by covering
the membrane sites on transformed cells with monovalent concanavalin A, Burger and Noonan (1970) restored the growth pattern of transformed fibroblasts to that of normal cells.

Apart from the increased agglutinability by plant lectins,
a number of other changes have been described in the surface
membranes of transformed cells. For instance, surface mucopoly-
saccharides are more strongly stained in electron micrographs of
transformed cells (Martinez-Palomo et al. 1969), and seven different glycosidases are increased after transformation of several
cell lines (Bosmann 1969). Sialyl-transferase, an enzyme involved

in sialic acid incorporation, is only half as active in transformed 3T3 cells than in untransformed ones (Grimes 1970), and so are other transglycolases (see review by Pardee 1971). There are exceptions, however, and, for instance, Van Beek et al. (1973) believe that increased sialylation of cell surface glycoproteins is characteristic of transformed cell lines (see Grimes 1974 for other exceptions).

Recently, numerous studies have described differences in the structure of the cell surface between normal and transformed cells, especially in relation to the fluidity of the cell membrane (Inbar et al. 1973), including clustering and mobility of lectin binding sites (Nicolson 1974, Sachs et. al. 1974). These differences have been critically discussed by Talmadge et al. (1974).

Most prominent, however, and better studied have been the changes in glycolipid and glycoprotein composition of the surface membranes of virally-transformed cells in culture. These vary from a decrease in transformed cells, in the content of sialic acid and galactosamine, to an increase in glucosamine content (Wu et al. 1969), to the absence of higher gangliosides in malignant cells (Hakomori 1970, Cumar et al. 1970). Differences between normal and transformed cells in surface labeling of galactosyl and galactosaminyl residues in surface glycoproteins and glycolipids, have been reported by Hakomori et al. (1974). According to Brady and Fishman (1974), the pattern of gangliosides is different in normal and tumorigenic cell lines, and the difference is primarily due to a decrease in the activity of hematoside: N-acetylgalactosaminyl-transferase which catalyzes an early step in the synthesis of the oligosaccharide chain of gangliosides. More convincing though are the investigations of Robbins and coworkers (Wickus et al. 1974). These authors used chick cells infected with TS-68, a mutant of the Schmidt-Ruppin strain of Rous sarcoma virus. Infected cells have the normal cell phenotype at 41° and the Rous transformed phenotype at 36°. Changes in the synthesis of the surface component proteins occur within 3 hours of induction of transformation by temperature shift. Related to Robbins' finding is the report of Hynes (1973) that a cell surface protein removed from "normal" NIL 8 cells by mild proteolytic digestion is absent or unavailable for iodination in virus-transformed cells. Similarly, a galactoprotein of M.W. ⁻ 200,000 is missing from the surface of transformed BHK cells (Gahmberg et al. 1974) or 3T3 cells (Hogg 1974). These changes in the anatomy of the cell membrane find functional support in the studies of Brailovsky et al. (1973) who reported that addition of glycolipids obtained from *Salmonella minnesota* R mutants to rat embryo fibroblasts in culture causes inhibition of growth of transformed cells but not of normal cells.

Finally, transport changes also occur in transformed cells. Foster and Pardee (1969) showed an approximately three-fold increase in uptake of certain amino acids by polyoma-transformed 3T3 cells as compared to the untransformed line. Hatanaka et al. (1970) have reported a dramatically lower Km value for glucose or mannose uptake in mouse cells transformed by a murine sarcoma virus.

While there is no question that the evidence for membrane changes in transformed cells is impressive, the conclusion that these changes might be responsible for uncontrolled growth is perhaps premature. There are several objections to this popular conclusion: (a) changes in agglutinability by plant lectins do not always correlate with saturation density, and especially with tumorigenicity (Grimes 1974); (b) the susceptibility to agglutination by concanavalin A and wheat germ agglutinin increases in chick embryo and in mammalian cells also when they are infected with nononcogenic viruses, such as Newcastle disease virus and Herpes simplex virus (Poste 1972); (c) similarly, increased mobility and redistribution of concanavalin A receptors can be caused by Newcastle disease virus (Poste and Reeve 1974); (d) covering concanavalin A binding sites on virally transformed cells with succinyl concanavalin A has no effect on their growth pattern (Trowbridge and Hilborn 1974); (e) transformed cells are not necessarily neoplastic and one should always remember Pontén's (1971) warning that ". . . the neoplastic or malignant potential of cells cannot be deduced without implanting cells into animals." In many experiments with transformed cells in culture, their transplantability into animals has not been verified; even brushing aside the above objections, the data reported in the literature are open to opposite interpretations, ie., they do not tell whether the changes are the cause or the effect of uncontrolled cell growth; (f) some of the changes, in fact, have been reported to occur in proliferating normal cells, which brings us directly into the second part of this chapter, namely, the functional and structural changes in cell membranes of proliferating cells during the cell cycle.

MEMBRANE CHANGES DURING THE CELL CYCLE

We have already discussed in a previous chapter the finding by Fox et al. (1971) that in normal 3T3 cells the wheat germ agglutinin-receptor site is exposed during a 1-hour period of their cell cycle, which coincides with mitosis. Significantly, the glycopeptides ephemerally expressed on the cell surface during mitosis are similar to those permanently expressed after viral transformation (Glick and Buck 1973). Other changes in the cell membrane occur during the cell cycle of dividing cells and these have been discussed in detail by Pardee (1971) in a previous review. Most of these changes are rather modest, with the exception of a change in electrophoretic mobility which, in sarcoma cells, also reaches a peak at mitosis. In CHO cells, just before mitosis there is a loss of surface heparin sulfate, a mucopolysaccharide similar to heparin (Kraemer and Tobey 1972). Synthesis of surface glycolipids during the cell cycle has been studied by Wolf and Robbins (1974). The majority of glycolipids are synthesized during all phases of the cell cycle, but two of them, called *GL-3* and *GL-4*, are preferentially synthesized during G_1 and early S. However, more important seem to be the changes that occur in cell membranes when proliferating cells cease to divide or when quiescent G_0 cells are stimulated to proliferate. Thus, Foster and Pardee (1969) demonstrated a small decrease in the transport of some amino acids when 3T3 cells are contact-inhibited. Numerous changes have been reported to occur in quiescent G_0 cells stimulated to proliferate. In fact Burger (1970) has reported, in a now classic

experiment, that brief treatment with trypsin or pronase causes
density-inhibited 3T3 mouse fibroblasts to resume growth. The
brief treatment with trypsin or pronase causes a change in the
cell membrane and, since normal fibroblasts repair their surface
damaged by trypsin treatment within 6 hours, they just go through
one round of cell division. However, even in this case there is a
lag period, a prereplicative phase, between the brief preteolytic
treatment and the onset of DNA synthesis and cell division. These
experiments by Burger are probably the most direct demonstration that changes in the cell surface can cause initiation of cell proliferation. It is interesting to note that stimulation of cell proliferation is not due to proteolytic activity of enzymes that have entered
the cell, since insoluble trypsin bound to beads was able to induce the
same phenomenon, even though all beads could be washed off the cell
surface after 5 minutes. These experiments, together with other experiments with sepharose-bound phytohemagglutinin, indicate that the
stimulation of cell proliferation in such cases may be caused by compounds acting directly on membranes without penetrating into the
cells.

An increased synthesis or turnover of membrane phospho-
lipids has been reported to occur in phytohemagglutinin-stimulated
lymphocytes (Kay 1968, Fisher and Mueller 1968), and in rodents
(Cunningham and Pardee 1971, Pasternak and Bergeron 1970) or
chick (Peterson and Rubin 1969) fibroblasts stimulated to proliferate. Changes in glycolipid synthesis have also been described in
resting NIL8 cells stimulated to proliferate (Critchley et al. 1974).
In L cells, instead, the turnover of various components of the cell
surface increases when exponentially growing cells become stationary (Warren and Glick 1968). However, the phenomenon that
has attracted the attention of most investigators is the increase in
transport function that takes place when stationary cells reenter
the proliferative cycle. The increase in transport function of low
molecular weight compounds (phosphate, nucleosides, amino
acids and so forth), is so regularly observed, that it has been construed as prima facie evidence for the primary role of surface
membranes in the regulation of cell proliferation. Table 9.1 gives
some illustrative examples, taken from the literature, of increased

transport function of cell membranes following a stimulus to
proliferate. As a brief digression we should remember that there
is more than one transport system, and that when we measure the
uptake of a compound we are only seeing one aspect of membrane
transport function. Thus, the transport of α-aminoisobutyric acid
into cells may depend on a transport system which promotes the
transport of proline and is different from the γ-glutamyltrans-
peptidase system that promotes transport of most other aminoacids (Meister 1973). Let us return to Table 9.1. The list is impressive and it tells us that an increase in membrane transport
function is an early event in the prereplicative phase of quiescent
cells stimulated to proliferate. In fact, in serum-stimulated 3T3
cells the increase in phosphate transport is instantaneous and
precedes the increase in uridine uptake and the decrease in the
intracellular concentration of cyclic AMP (De Asua et al. 1974).
Current dogma also states that the increase in transport function
is *the* triggering event, which sets in motion all other biochemical
changes leading to DNA synthesis and cell division. But a number
of observations in the literature seem to refuse the constraints
of the dogma. These observations include: (a) in WI-38, in rat
uterus, and in isoleucine deprived CHO cells, the increase in membrane transport function occurs relatively late in the prereplicative
phase, certainly after several events (gene activation, increased
synthesis of nonhistone chromosomal proteins) have already
taken place. Incidentally, if one is allowed an incursion in the
related field of gene expression, we should remember that the appearance of 1α, 25-dihydroxycholecalciferol specifically bound to
chromatin of intestinal mucosa precedes the increase in calcium
absorption by 2-8 hours (Brumbaugh and Haussler 1974). (b) The
behavior of CHO cells (prompt increase when mitotic cells go into
G_1, delayed increase when stationary cells are stimulated to proliferate) seems to suggest that the increase in membrane transport
function in G_0 cells is secondary to other events (see also chapter
11 on G_0 vs G_1 cells). (c) Estrogens, while stimulating cell growth,
do not apparently interact with cell membranes. In mammalian
target tissues they combine directly with a cytoplasmic protein
(Toft and Gorski 1966) without any detectable effect on mem-

Table 9.1   Changes in Membrane Transport Function Occurring in Stationary Cells Stimulated to Proliferate[a]

Cell type	Stimulus	Compound(s) tested	Time[b] (hr)	Reference
3T3	Serum	Phosphate	<0.01	DeAsua et al. (1974)
3T3	Serum	Uridine	0.15	DeAsua et al. (1974)
3T3	Serum	Uridine phosphate	0.25	Cunningham and Pardee (1969)
Chick fibroblasts	Serum or trypsin	2-deoxyglucose	0.25	Sefton and Rubin (1971)
WI-38 fibroblasts	Serum	Leucine	3.0	Rovera and Baserga (1971)
WI-38 fibroblasts	Serum	Cycloleucine	3.0	Costlow and Baserga (1973)
3T6	Serum	Cycloleucine	1.0	Costolow and Baserga (1973)
2RA	Serum	Cycloleucine	1.0	Costlow and Baserga (1973)
CHO	c	2-Aminoisobutyric acid	1.0	Sander and Pardee (1972)
CHO	d	2-Aminoisobutyric acid	3.0	Sander and Pardee (1972)
Lymphocytes	Phytohemagglutinin	2-Aminoisobutyric acid	0.75	Medelsohn et al. (1971)
Lymphocytes	Concanavalin A	2-Aminoisobutyric acid	1.0	Van den Berg and Betel (1974)
Uterus (rat)	Estrogens	Uridine	2.0	Billing et al. (1969)

[a] Except for the rat uterus, all other systems listed in this Table are cells in culture. In all cases, the change in function is an *increase* in uptake of the compound tested.

[b] Earliest time (after stimulation) in which an increase could be detected.

[c] Mitotic cells mechanically detached and continuing directly into G_1.

[d] Cells made stationary by isoleucine-deprivation and stimulated by addition of isoleucine.

branes and from there they proceed to the nucleus where they
cause biochemical events (Glasser et al. 1972) which clearly precede the increase in membrane transport function cited in Table
9.1. In chick liver (another target tissue) estrogens interact directly with nuclear components (Lebeau et al. 1973). (d) There
is a dissociation between growth factors that stimulate cell proliferation and factors that stimulate uptake of low molecular
weight compounds. Thus, the serum fraction that stimulates uptake is different from the fraction that stimulates proliferation in
3T3 cells (Cunningham and Pardee 1969, 1971), and the factors
from conditioned medium that promote growth in BHK cells
are heat-labile, while the factors that increase uptake of non-
metabolizable amino acids are heat-stable (Shodell and Isselbacher
1973). (e) In some cases, as in concanavalin A-stimulated rat
lymphocytes, the early increase in the transport rate of amino-
isobutyric acid is inhibited by cycloheximide or puromycin
(Van den Berg and Betel 1974), which suggest events preceding
the membrane changes. (f) The stimulatory effect of proteases
on cell proliferation seems to be dissociated from its effect on
membranes. Thus, trypsin or pronase do not cause stimulation
of cell proliferation in confluent monolayers of WI-38 fibroblasts
(unless the cells are replated at a lower density), and the calf
serum fraction that promotes growth in chick embryo fibroblasts
not only has no protease activity, but is actually an inhibitor of
trypsin (Pierson and Temin 1972). Even more definite is the report
of Glynn et al. (1973) that pronase sometimes fails to stimulate
3T3 cells to proliferate and yet produces the characteristic membrane changes.

What, then, are the conclusions? First of all there is no
doubt that membrane changes (functional and structural) occur
in cells stimulated to proliferate and in transformed cells that
have lost density-dependent inhibition of growth. The question
is, are these changes the cause or the effect of cell proliferation?
The evidence presented in this chapter seems to indicate that
membrane changes may actually be secondary to other events occurring within the cell in response to external stimuli. The only

exception would be the increase in phosphate uptake that occurs immediately after serum is added to cultures of 3T3 cells (De Asua et al. 1974), but there is no evidence yet that this increase is correlated to the stimulation of cell proliferation. It could simply represent a serum effect, distinct from the ability of serum to stimulate cell proliferation, as suggested by the experiments of Cunningham and Pardee (1969). While it is true that in some cases (trypsin and 3T3 cells) the proliferative stimulus may act directly on the membrane, this is not a requirement (for instance, estrogens), and a plausible explanation of the data reported in the literature is that the stimuli (with or without the intermediary of the cell membrane) cause a change within the cell, which, in turn, sets in motion the chain of biochemical events, including membrane changes, eventually leading to DNA synthesis and cell division.

This, of course, is rank heresy and the good Dominicans of membrane supremacy will retort that undetected membrane changes may occur immediately after stimulation, before any other biochemical event, which brings us back to the old Augustinian prob-problem of the superiority of revelation over reason.

We have now come to the end of our story after examining in detail the various biochemical events that occur in dividing cells and in cells stimulated to proliferate. We will summarize the situation in chapter 13, where we will also try to understand the problem of the cancer cell in light of the working hypothesis for the control of cell proliferation in mammalian cells that can be built upon the findings thus far described. Before this, though, let us consider a few related topics.

References

Abercrombie, M. and Ambrose, E.J. (1962). *Cancer Res. 22*: 525-548.
van Beek, W.P., Smets, L.A., and Emmelot, P. (1973). *Cancer Res. 33*: 2913-2922.
Billing, E.J., Barbiroli, B., and Smellie, R.M.S. (1969). *Biochim. Biophys. Acta 190*: 52-59.

Bosmann, H.B. (1969). *Exp. Cell Res. 54*: 217-221.

Brady, R.O. and Fishman, P.H. (1974). In *Control of Proliferation in Animal Cells,* B. Clarkson and R. Baserga (Eds.). Cold Spring Harbor Laboratory, pp. 505-515.

Brailovsky, C., Trudel, M., Lallier, R., and Nigam, V.N. (1973). *J. Cell Biol. 57*: 124-132.

Brumbaugh, P.F. and Haussler, M.R. (1974). *J. Biol. Chem. 249*: 1251-1257.

Burger, M.M. (1969). *Proc. Natl. Acad. Sci. USA 62*: 994-1001.

Burger, M.M. (1970). *Nature 227*: 170-171.

Burger, M.M. (1971). *Nature New Biol. 231*: 512-515.

Burger, M.M. (1972). In *Biomembranes vol. 2* L. Manson (Ed.). 247-270.

Burger, M.M. and Noonan, K.D. (1970). *Nature 228*: 512-515.

Costlow, M. and Baserga, R. (1973). *J. Cell. Physiol. 82*: 411-419.

Critchley, D.R., Chandrabose, K.A., Graham, J.M., and MacPherson, I. (1974). In *Control of Proliferation in Animal Cells,* B. Clarkson and R. Baserga (Eds.). Cold Spring Harbor Laboratory, pp. 481-493.

Cumar, F.A., Brady, R.O., Kolodny, E.H., McFarland, V.W., and Mora, P.T. (1970). *Proc. Natl. Acad. Sci. USA 67*: 757-764.

Cunningham, D.D. and Pardee, A.B. (1969). *Proc. Natl. Acad. Sci. USA 64*: 1049-1056.

Cunningham, D.D. and Pardee, A.B. (1971). In *Ciba Symposium,* G.E.W. Wolstenholme and Julie Knight (Eds.). *On Growth Control in Cell Cultures.* Churchill-Livingstone, London, pp. 207-220.

DeAsua, L.J., Rozengurt, E., and Dulbecco, R. (1974). *Proc. Natl. Acad. Sci. USA 71*: 96-98.

Eckhart, W., Dulbecco, R., and Burger, M.M. (1971). *Proc. Natl. Acad. Sci. USA 68*: 283-286.

Fisher, D.B. and Mueller, G.C. (1968). *Proc. Natl. Acad. Sci. USA 60*: 1396-1402.

Foster, D.O. and Pardee, A.B. (1969). *J. Biol. Chem. 244*: 2675-2681.

Fox, T.O., Shephard, J.R., and Burger, M.M. (1971). *Proc. Natl. Acad. Sci. USA 68*: 244-247.

Gahmberg, C.G., Kiehn, D., and Hakomori, S. (1974). *Nature 248*: 413-415.

Glasser, S.R., Chytil, F., and Spelsberg, T.C. (1972). *Biochem. J. 130*: 947-957.

Glick, M.C. and Buck, C.A. (1973). *Biochemistry 12*: 85-90.

Glynn, R.D., Thrash, C.R., and Cunningham, D.D. (1973). *Proc. Natl. Acad. Sci. USA 70*: 2676-2677.

Grimes, W.J. (1970). *Biochemistry 9*: 5083-5092.

Grimes, W.J. (1974). In *Control of Proliferation in Animal Cells,* B. Clarkson and R. Baserga (Eds.). Cold Spring Harbor Laboratory, pp. 517-531.

Hakomori, S. (1970). *Proc. Natl. Acad. Sci. USA* 67: 1741-1747.

Hakomori, S., Teather, C., and Andrews, H. (1968). *Biochem. Biophys. Res. Comm. 33*: 563-568.

Hakomori, S., Gahmberg, C.G., Laine, R., and Kijimoto, S. (1974). In *Control of Proliferation in Animal Cells,* B. Clarkson and R. Baserga (Eds.). Cold Spring Harbor Laboratory, pp. 461-471.

Hatanaka, M., Huebner, R.J., and Gilden, R.V. (1970). *J. Natl. Canc. Inst. 43*: 1091-1096.

Hayry, P. and Defendi, V. (1970). *Virology 41*: 22-29.

Hogg, N.M. (1974). *Proc. Natl. Acad. Sci. USA 71*: 489-492.

Hynes, R.O. (1973). *Proc. Natl. Acad. Sci. USA 70*: 3170-3174.

Inbar, M., Ben-Bassat, H., Fibach, E., and Sachs, L. (1973). *Proc. Natl. Acad. Sci. USA 70*: 2577-2581.

Inbar, M. and Sachs, L. (1969). *Proc. Natl. Acad. Sci. USA 63*: 1418-1425.

Kay, J.E. (1968). *Nature 219*: 172-173.

Kraemer, P.M. and Tobey, R.A. (1972). *J. Cell. Biol. 55*: 713-717.

Lebeau, M., Massol, N., and Baulie, E. (1973). *Eur. J. Biochem. 36*: 294-300.

Martinez-Palomo, A., Brailovsky, C., and Bernhard, W. (1969). *Cancer Res. 29*: 925-937.

Meister, A. (1973). *Science 180*: 33-39.

Mendelsohn, J., Skinner, A., and Kornfeld, S. (1971). *J. Clin. Invest. 50*: 818-826.

Nicolson, G.L. (1974). In *Control of Proliferation in Animal Cells,* B. Clarkson and R. Baserga (Eds.). Cold Spring Harbor Laboratory, pp. 251-270.

Pardee, A.B. (1964). *Natl. Canc. Inst. Monogr. 14*: 7-18.

Pardee, A.B. (1971). *In Vitro 7*: 95-104.

Pasternak, C.A. and Bergeron, J.J.M. (1970). *Biochem. J. 119*: 473-480.

Peterson, J.A. and Rubin, H. (1969). *Exp. Cell Res. 58*: 365-378.

Pierson, R.W. Jr. and Temin, H.M. (1972). *J. Cell. Physiol. 79*: 319-330.

Pontén, J. (1971). *Spontaneous and Virus Induced Transformation in Cell Culture.* Springer-Verlag, New York, pp. 8-15.

Poste, G. (1972). *Exp. Cell Res. 73*: 319-328.

Poste, G. and Reeve, P. (1974). *Nature 247*: 469-471.

Rovera, G. and Baserga, R. (1971). *J. Cell. Physiol. 77*: 201-212.

Sachs, L., Inbar, M., and Shinitzky, M. (1974). In *Control of Proliferation in Animal Cells,* B. Clarkson and R. Baserga (Eds.). Cold Spring Harbor Laboratory, pp. 283-296.

Sander, G. and Pardee, A.B. (1972). *J. Cell Physiol. 80*: 267-272.

Sefton, B.M. and Rubin, H. (1971). *Proc. Natl. Acad. Sci. USA 68*: 3154-3157.

Shodell, M. and Isselbacher, K. (1973). *Nature New Biol. 243*: 83-85.

Stoker, M.G.P. (1969). In *Homeostatic Regulators,* G.E.W. Wolstenholme and J. Knight (Eds.). J. & A. Churchill, Ltd., London, pp. 264-271.

Talmadge, K.W., Noonan, K.D., and Burger, M.M. (1974). In *Control of Proliferation in Animal Cells,* B. Clarkson and R. Baserga (Eds.). Cold Spring Harbor Laboratory, pp. 313-325.

Toft, D. and Gorski, J. (1966). *Proc. Natl. Acad. Sci. USA 55*: 1574-1581.

Trowbridge, I.S. and Hilborn, D.A. (1974). *Nature 250*: 304-307.

Van den Berg, K.J. and Betel, I. (1974). *Exp. Cell Res. 84*: 412-418.

Warren, L. and Glick, M.C. (1968). *J. Cell Biol. 37*: 729-746.

Weber, J.J. (1973). *J. Cell. Physiol. 81*: 49-53.

Wickus, G.G., Branton, P.E., and Robbins, P.W. (1974). In *Control of Proliferation in Animal Cells,* B. Clarkson and R. Baserga (Eds.). Cold Spring Harbor Laboratory, pp. 541-546.

Wolf, B.A. and Robbins, P.W. (1974). In *Control of Proliferation in Animal Cells,* B. Clarkson and R. Baserga (Eds.). pp. 473-479.

Wu., H.C., Meezan, E., Black, P.H., and Robbins, P.W. (1969). *Biochemistry 8*: 2509-2517.

TEN

GROWTH FACTORS

DEFINITION OF GROWTH FACTORS

A monograph of this kind would not be complete without a discussion of growth factors. Unfortunately, an adequate discussion of the factors that have been reported to regulate cell proliferation in man, in experimental animals, and in cell cultures would require a book by itself. Furthermore, a critical analysis of growth factors involves problems of considerable magnitude. Here are listed a few of these problems, just to give the reader an idea of the difficulties one faces when trying to put some order in this confusion:

1. Are growth factors active in cell cultures relevant to the regulation of cell proliferation in animals? While there are instances in which growth factors active in cell cultures seem, indeed, to be identical with those involved in the control of cell proliferation and differentiation in animals, there are other instances in which growth factors for cells in culture have obviously little to do with the control of cell proliferation in animals. In between a few clear-cut instances, there are many others in which a decision one way or the other can not be made at the present moment.

2. What should we consider among growth factors? The fundamental work of Eagle (1955) has established, a long time ago, that

cells in culture require certain nutrients for proper maintenance and growth (for the history and composition of synthetic media see review by Waymouth 1965). If one were to include among growth factors the amino acids, vitamins, and other nutrients that make up Eagle's medium and proceed to a detailed discussion of them, one would be faced with the task of compiling a text book or two of biochemistry and nutrition. The same comments apply to the pH of cultures. Again Eagle and his collaborators (Eagle 1973) recently reemphasized the importance of pH in regulating the growth of cells in culture (is that the shadow of Claude Bernard that I see smiling in Hades?). Still, I do not believe that pH should be included among growth factors.

3. The problem of defining a growth factor is by no means peculiar to cells in culture. For instance, we have repeatedly seen in this monograph that the acinar cells of mouse salivary glands can be stimulated to synthesize DNA and divide by a synthetic catecholamine, isoproterenol. As fond of this model as I have been in past years, by no stretch of imagination would I pretend that isoproterenol is the physiological regulator of cell proliferation in salivary glands of rodents.

4. As we shall see later, growth factors may be tissue specific and species specific. Thus, a factor that may be necessary for growth of a certain type of cells in culture may be totally indifferent or even harmful to other types of cells, which is another way of translating that Japanese haiku "the grass the cow eats turns into milk, the grass the snake eats turns into poison."

5. Growth factors can be divided into those that stimulate and those that inhibit cell growth. Stimulatory factors, because they display a positive action, are slightly less likely to be artifactual than inhibitory factors, where the credibility gap is considerable. It is indeed quite easy to inhibit cell proliferation with a variety of drugs and chemicals, most of which have nothing to do with the physiological control of cell division. Even macromolecules that have an inhibitory action on cell cultures can be totally artifactual. For instance, a few years ago it was found that a

protein isolated from rat liver and that bound certain chemical carcinogens, inhibited the growth of cells in culture. Although the findings were scientifically correct, it turned out eventually that the protein was arginase, which by merrily catobolizing one of the amino acids required by cells in culture, caused aspecific inhibition of cell proliferation and death.

6. Even when we limit ourselves to stimulatory growth factors, we must make a distinction between factors that control the saturation density of newly plated cells, those that will stimulate cell proliferation in quiescent confluent monolayers, and those necessary for cell survival. Although some of the factors may display all three properties, other have unique activities, as already apparent from published reports (Paul et al. 1971).

These are just a few of the problems that one has to face in a discussion of growth factors. I hope, therefore, that the reader will bear with me if I make an arbitrary selection and concentrate on those macromolecular factors that seem to offer the best promise as possible candidates for the physiological regulation of cell division. Hormones in animals will not be listed among growth factors, although their role is exquisitely physiological. And with these premises, let us begin by dividing growth factors into stimulatory and inhibitory and into factors that affect cells in culture and factors that affect cells in animals.

STIMULATORY FACTORS IN CELL CULTURES

It has been known for a long time that the chemically undefined entity called serum is necessary for the growth of cells in culture. Although a few cell lines have been reported to grow in chemically defined media (Waymouth 1965), the great majority of cell lines require a certain amount of serum. In fact, it has been customary to consider normal those cells that have stringent requirements for a relatively high concentration of serum (Holley and Kiernan 1968, Jainchill and Todaro, 1970) and transformed those that need smaller amounts (see several papers in the Wistar Institute Monograph edited by Defendi and Stoker 1967, also see Kruse et al. 1969). Ponten (1971) and others have considered this problem in detail, and the common conclusion is that serum requirements are more stringent for normal than for transformed cells. Unfortunately, as Westermark (1973) pointed out, investigators have often taken as the virtuous model of normal cells, 3T3 cells, which are aneuploid cells with a low saturation density. Westermark (1973) considers 3T3 cells, and similar cell lines, as "pseudonormal" and believes that diploid cells should serve as the normal counterpart for comparison with transformed cells. He points out that pseudonormal cells, such as 3T3 mouse cells and BHK hamster cells, cannot be regarded as ideal controls because they are heteroploid and genetically unstable. In addition, the capacity to undergo an unlimited number of divisions is a deviation from normal nonhematopoietic cell behavior (Ponten 1971). However, even when diploid cells, such as WI-38 human diploid fibroblasts or the glia-like cells used by Westermark (1973) are taken as proper controls, it is apparent that normal cells have a requirement for serum which largely exceeds the requirements of transformed cell lines.

Holley and Kiernan (1968) were the first ones to quantitatively demonstrate that the concentration of serum determined the final saturation density even of low-saturation density cell lines such as 3T3 mouse cells. That the saturation density is dependent upon the supply of available medium had already been shown by Stoker and Rubin (1967) and by Kruse and Miedema (1965) who, using the technique of continuous perfusion, grew WI-38 human diploid fibroblasts into layers 5-6 cells thick. However, more recently, Oey et al (1974) proposed that growth control in cultured fibroblasts is mediated through both density-specific and serum-specific regulations, which can be independent and separate entities. For instance, sensitivity to serum restriction, but not sensitivity to density-restriction, is accompanied by a greatly increased intracellular concentration of cyclic AMP. Returning to serum, numerous attempts have been carried out to isolate the substance, or substances, from serum responsible for the growth

control of cells in culture. The results are, to say the least, contradictory. Thus a number of investigators in Holley's laboratory
have identified several fractions necessary for the maintenance
and growth of either 3T3 cells or their SV-40 transformed counterparts (Paul et al. 1971). The factors, however, are multiple (Holley
1974), and the sum of the factors never equals the efficacy of
unfractionated serum itself. Jainchill and Todaro (1970) reported
that agamma serum, ie., serum without the gamma globulin
fraction, is devoid of growth stimulatory properties for 3T3 cells,
but the results have never been confirmed and there are lingering
doubts about their reproducibility. To complicate matters, Houck
and Cheng (1973) and Hoffman et al. (1973), isolated fractions
from calf serum which, according to them, have the total activity
of serum in regulating growth of cells in culture. From mammalian
serum, Houck and Cheng (1973) isolated and purified a single
sialoprotein, with a molecular weight of 120,000, that can quantitatively replace serum in supporting growth of WI-38 human
diploid fibroblasts. On the other hand, using rat fibroblasts as
the test cells, Hoffman et al. (1973) isolated two separate proteins with molecular weights of 26,000 and $>$ 600,000, respectively.
Both proteins, which were isolated from fetal calf serum, must
be present to stimulate growth. Another serum protein that,
according to Ellem and Mironescu (1972), can replace serum in
stimulating human diploid fibroblasts, is albumin. But Bates and
Levene (1970), using 3T6 cells, found that the albumin-containing
fraction of serum was so devoid of growth-promoting activity
that they used it as a control for the physical effects of proteins
in the absence of serum. This is confusion elevated to art. The
best one can do in such circumstances is to say that serum is one
of the growth factors required for cells in culture and that different cells may utilize different factors from each kind of serum,
and leave it at that.

A number of growth stimulatory factors have been reported in the literature and some of these are listed in Table 10.1,
together with the test cells, because, as mentioned above, many

TABLE 10.1 **Growth Stimulatory Factors in Cell Cultures**

Cell type	Factor	References
3T3 mouse fibroblasts	Serum	Holley and Kiernan (1968)
3T3 mouse fibroblasts	FGF	Gospodarowicz (1974)
3T3 mouse fibroblasts	Trypsin	Burger (1970)
3T6 mouse fibroblasts	Serum	Bates and Levene (1973)
WI-38 human diploid fibroblasts	Sialoprotein from serum	Houck and Cheng (1973)
Rat fibroblasts	Two proteins from serum	Hoffman et al. (1973)
Chick embryo cells	Insulin, neuraminidase trypsin, papain	Vaheri et al. (1973)
Amnion cells	Hydrocortisone	Connor and Marti (1966)
Chick embryo fibroblasts	MSA	Dulak and Temin (1973)
Fetal rat hepatocytes	Serum (ornithine, arginine)	Paul and Walter (1974)
BHK	Conditioned medium	Shodell and Isselbacher (1973)
Mouse macrophage	MGF	Mauel and Defendi (1971)
Pancreatic epithelia	Mesenchymal factor	Levine et al. (1973)
Granulocytes	Colony-stimulating factor	Metcalf (1971)
Epidermal cells	Epidermal growth factor	Cohen (1962)
Nerve cells	Nerve growth factor	Levi-Montalcini (1966)
Neoplastic liver cells	A tripeptide	Pickart and Thaler (1973)

of these factors are tissue-and species-specific and have a very limited range of action. Typical of this is the effect of certain stimulatory factors like trypsin, neuraminidase, insulin, hydrocortisone, and others. Most of these compounds are effective on chick fibroblasts and occasionally on mouse fibroblasts, but are ineffective in stimulating growth in human fibroblasts. An interesting growth factor is the polypeptide isolated from brain and pituitary and called FGF by Gospodarowicz (1974), which

stimulates cell proliferation in quiescent 3T3 cells and whose
action is potentiated by hydrocortisone. It is a good example of
a growth factor that is very likely to have a physiological role
in animals. At the opposite end are the findings of Paul and Walter
(1974) that arginine or ornithine can induce DNA synthesis (in the
presence of serum) in rat hepatocytes. The possibility that these
two amino acids may play some part in regulating growth of liver
cells is remote.

Apart from the serum proteins isolated by Houck and
Cheng (1973) and by Hoffman et al. (1973), one of the stimulatory growth factors that has been better studied is a partially purified polypeptide fraction isolated from serum-free medium conditioned by rat cells. This partially purified fraction, which has many
characteristics in common with somatomedin (Hall and Uthne
1971), supports, but not quantitatively, the growth of chicken and
rat embryo fibroblasts (Dulak and Temin 1973). It has been called
MSA, it has a nonsuppressible insulin-like activity, and it is not
only devoid of protease activity but it actually inhibits trypsin
(Pierson and Temin 1972). It should be noted at this point that,
although the stimulatory activities of insulin and serum can often
go together, it is possible to separate from serum a factor that
stimulates DNA synthesis from a factor that has insulin-like
activity (Scher et al. 1974).

Other factors have been isolated from conditioned
medium and are known to stimulate the growth of certain cells.
For instance, factors have been isolated from medium conditioned
by L-mouse cells that stimulate division in macrophages (Mauel and
Defendi 1971) or in BHK cells (Shodell and Isselbacher 1973). There
are also cell-specific, reasonably purified factors that affect both
cell proliferation and differentiation, for example, those of Levine
et al. (1973) and some of the factors described for hemopoietic
tissues (see review by Metcalf 1971 and more recent papers by Till
et al. 1974 and Sachs 1974). However, cell proliferation is complicated enough without tackling the problem of cell differentiation, which we shall avoid in this monograph. Some of the growth

regulatory factors reported in the literature have been omitted from our table because they have been found to be artifactual. In fact, if the reader wishes to fully appreciate the ephemeral life of growth factors, he should consult three references that are only a few years apart. The first one is a symposium held at the Wistar Institute and edited in 1967 by Defendi and Stoker. The second one is a Ciba Foundation Symposium (Wolstenholme and Knight) published in 1969 and, the third one is a Symposium on Control of Proliferation in Animal Cells that was held at Cold Spring Harbor and published in 1974 (Clarkson and Baserga). A comparison of these three references will convince even the most skeptical reader of the rapidly changing picture of growth factors and of the short half-life that many of these factors have.

STIMULATORY FACTORS IN ANIMALS

If we include hormones, such as estrogens, progesterone, and growth hormone, very little is known about growth factors that stimulate cell proliferation in *corpore vile*. Most of our knowledge comes from studies on regenerating liver. For several years investigators have been trying to identify and isolate the growth factor that promotes proliferation of liver cells after partial hepatectomy. Complicated cross-transfusion experiments have been devised for this purpose, and despite some contradictory results the evidence seems to favor the possibility that a circulating growth factor in serum may trigger cell proliferation in the remaining liver cells (Bucher et al. 1969). In my opinion, better evidence, at least from a biological point of view, has come from experiments in which a partial hepatectomy was performed on animals bearing transplants of normal liver or of well-differentiated hepatomas. Leong et al. (1964) showed that when partial hepatectomy is performed in a rat carrying a subcutaneous liver graft, cell proliferation is induced in the hepatocytes of the graft. In similar experiments Lee (1971) has shown stimulation of cell proliferation in subcutaneously growing hepatomas of rats after partial

hepatectomy. These experiments not only indicate the presence of
a diffusible factor in partial hepatectomized animals that may
stimulate proliferation of liver cells, but they also offer the possibility of some elegant experiments on remote controls.

Another interesting experimental manipulation was recently reported by Short et al. (1973), in rats on a protein-free
diet for 3 days and without food for 8 hours that were given
protein-containing food ad libitum. In these rats the incorporation
of thymidine ^{3}H into liver cells DNA increased, beginning at 8
hours, and reached a peak at 16 hours when it was about tenfold
the control levels. The most effective procedure was to feed rats
after the starvation period with a diet containing 60% proteins.
Lee et al. (1968) also showed that a single injection of tri-
iodothyronine causes timulation of DNA synthesis and cell division
in rat liver. These findings were subsequently confirmed by Short
et al. (1972) who found that a mixture of tri-iodothyronine, glucagon,
heparin, and amino acids was effective in stimulating DNA synthesis
in liver cells. Isoleucine, threonine, and valine were found to be the
only three amino acids essential for the increase in DNA synthesis
(Short et al. 1974). However, with these experiments we are again
entering the field of hormones and nutrition, which, as mentioned
above, constitute a story in themselves. For the moment all that
can be said is that very little information is available on diffusible
macromolecular factors that may regulate cell proliferation in
animals.

INHIBITORY FACTORS

Macromolecular factors capable of inhibiting the growth
of cells in culture, or in the growing animal, have been described for
a number of years. We have already mentioned that most of these
factors must be disqualified from the list of growth factors because
they are totally nonspecific and act purely by starving cells of essential
nutritional requirements or by killing them. Thus, as a first rule for

the diplomatic recognition of an inhibitory factor, I would like to propose that it must be capable of arresting cells at some specific point of the cell cycle. For instance, protease inhibitors do not stop cells at some specific point of the cell's life cycle and are therefore not considered as growth inhibitors (Schnebli and Haemmerli 1974). This definition would eliminate many candidates. However, after the dust has settled and a great number of claims are disposed of, there are still a number of inhibitory factors that deserve our attention as possible regulatory mechanisms of cell proliferation. Most popular among these inhibitory factors are certainly those substances called *chalones*, a term introduced several years ago by Bullough and Laurence (1960). A brief digression on a personal matter is in order at this point. On a number of occasions, colleagues have informed me that I enjoy the reputation (or the notoriety, depending on the point of view) of being "against chalones." *Est auctor quis denique eorum vixi cum quibus*? I have never questioned the existence of inhibitory growth factors, either in cell cultures or in animals. The problem with chalones is that they have been successively described as substances of low molecular weight, high molecular weight, thermostabile, thermolabile, tissue specific, aspecific, and so on. Too many and varied compounds have been listed under the name of chalones, which could do nothing else but discredit the name itself to the point that one would find it difficult to argue with the statement of Rutter et al. (1973) that "specific feedback inhibitors (chalones) have been poorly documented and, in most cases, seem more a conceptual possibility than an experimentally documented fact." However, if we remove from the term *chalone* some of the extravagant claims that have been made in its name, one is still left with an interesting list of inhibitory growth factors. The reader who wishes to know more about chalones is referred to a recent review by Houck and Hennings (1973). According to these authors chalones are characterized by: (a) cell-specificity; (b) lack of species-specificity; and (c) reversibility, and the evidence for their existence is most convincing for four chalone systems: epidermis, melanocyte, fibroblast, and lymphocyte. The uncertainties that still exist, for in-

stance, the epidermal chalone, are best exemplified by a recent
review written by one of its discoverers (Laurence 1973). To
quote from Laurence's review, ". . . there is considerable discrepancy
between results from in vitro experiments and from those performed
in vivo. Also, the various extracts from different laboratories are
not identical and even may not be chalones." Notwithstanding the
overgrowth of reports, it is possible to divide chalones into those
that act in G_1 and those that act in G_2. A typical example of a G_1
chalone is the liver chalone reported by Simard et al. (1974), which
inhibits the $G_1 \rightarrow$ S transition in proliferating liver cells. In most
cases they have not been purified to any reasonable extent, but
Houck and coworkers (1972) reported a protein of molecular
weight between 30,000 and 50,000 isolated from human diploid
fibroblasts that specifically inhibit the proliferation of human
diploid fibroblasts. In a subsequent study, Houck et al. (1973)
showed that the fibroblastic chalone inhibits the stimulatory effect of human fibroblasts by the serum sialoprotein mentioned
above among stimulatory growth factors. This, of course, would be
an extremely interesting problem, but its existence has not yet been
confirmed. The same problem seems to face another inhibitory
factor that was originally reported by Yeh and Fisher (1969) who
isolated a diffusible factor that sustained the state of contact-inhibition in confluent 3T3 cultures. To the category of chalones
also belongs a protein produced by and isolated from a contact-
inhibited melanocytic cell line, which is capable of restoring contact-
inhibition of cell division to highly malignant hamster melanocytes
(Lipkin and Knecht 1974). If confirmed, this finding would bring
chalones into the realm of practical applications.

MECHANISM OF INHIBITION

Despite the obvious problems inherent with the isolation and purification of inhibitory growth factors, the various
macromolecular factors listed above are still of considerable interest,
if nothing else, as possible experimental models for a thorough

search for inhibitory factors. Indeed, an analysis of growth in animals and in cells in culture seems to indicate, as a reasonable explanation, the accumulation of a growth inhibitory factor, causing
cell proliferation to cease once it reaches a critical concentration.
This factor does not necessarily have to be present in the intercellular fluid or medium. There have been several interesting reports
in the literature indicating that proteins with a respectable molecular weight (even up to 60,000) can pass directly from one cell to
another. A good review of membrane junctions in growth and differentiation, with the discussion of cell-to-cell flow of molecules
up to the order of 10,000 in molecular weight, can be found in
Loewenstein (1973). However, a more specific example has been
reported by Kolodny (1973) who, using 3T3 cells, showed that
histones and other nuclear proteins as well as cytoplasmic proteins,
are transferred from one cell to another without leaking out into
the medium. That contact between cells is not responsible per
se for the cessation of cell division has become increasingly apparent in recent years. The experiments of Holley and Kiernan (1968)
and more recently those of Dulbecco and Elkington (1973) and of
Stoker (1973) have shown that the availability of serum and nutrients,
and not cell-to-cell contact, determine the saturation density of
fibroblasts. Dulbecco and Elkington (1973) have indeed stated
that ". . . there is no experimental support for the concept that
contact inhibition of growth is responsible for cessation of
growth in dense cultures." However, contact between cells may
facilitate the diffusion of an inhibitory growth factor whose production or activation may be adversely influenced by serum or
other nutrients.

It is therefore possible that inhibitory factors may accumulate inside cells and, through membrane junctions, diffuse
from one cell to another and cause, when they reach a critical
concentration, cessation of cell proliferation. These factors ought
to be tissue specific since cells of other types are usually not affected by restrictions in cell proliferation occurring in one cell
type.

In conclusion, as a tentative picture in this very confused topic I would like to propose, for the reader's consideration, a model in which growth inhibitory factors determine the cessation of cell proliferation by diffusion from one cell to another, more likely through direct contact than through the intermediary of extracellular fluid. Cell proliferation resumes when a stimulatory factor is produced or furnished from the outside to counteract the inhibitory macromolecular factor. Although this is purely speculative, it is no more speculative than most of the factors that have been reported thus far and may, at least, offer some guidelines for studying the mysterious substances that have charmed and betrayed investigators for so many years.

References

Bates, C.J. and Levene, C.I. (1970) *J. Cell Sci.* 7: 683-693.
Bucher, N., Swaffield, M., Moolten, F., and Schrock, T. (1969). In *Biochemistry of Cell Division,* R. Baserga (Ed.). Charles C. Thomas, Springfield, Ill., pp. 139-154.
Bullough, W.S. and Laurence, E.B. (1960). *Proc. R. Soc. B. 151*: 517-536.
Burger, M.M. (1970). *Nature 227*: 170-171.
Clarkson, B. and Baserga. R. (Eds). *Control of Proliferation in Animal Cells.* Cold Spring Harbor Laboratory, 1974, Passim.
Cohen, S. (1962). *J. Biol. Chem. 237*: 1555-1562.
Connor, J.D. and Marti, A. (1966). *Proc. Soc. Exp. Biol. Med. 123*: 730-735.
Defendi, V. and Stoker, M. (Eds.). *Growth Regulating Substances for Animal Cells in Culture.* Wistar Inst. Press, Philadelphia, 1967, passim.
Dulak, N.C. and Temin, H.M. (1973). *J. Cell. Physiol. 81*: 153-160.
Dulbecco, R. and Elkington, J. (1973). *Nature 246*: 197-199.
Eagle, H. (1955). *Science 122*: 501-504.
Eagle, H. (1973). *J. Cell. Physiol. 82*: 1-8.
Ellem, K.A.O. and Mironescu, S. (1972). *J. Cell. Physiol. 79*: 389-406.
Gospodarowicz, D. (1974). *Nature 249*: 123-127.
Hall, K. and Uthne, K. (1971). *Acta Med. Scand. 190*: 137-143.
Hoffman, R., Ristow, H.J., Vesser, J., and Frank, W. (1973). *Exp. Cell Res. 85*: 275-280.

Holley, R.W. (1974). In *Control of Proliferation in Animal Cells*, B. Clarkson and R. Baserga (Eds.). Cold Spring Harbor Laboratory, pp. 13-18.

Holley, R.W. and Kiernan, J.A. (1968). *Proc. Natl. Acad. Sci. USA 60*: 300-304.

Houck, J.C. and Cheng, R.F. (1973). *J. Cell. Physiol. 81*: 257-270.

Houck, J.C. and Hennings, H. (1973). *FEBS Letters 32*: 1-8.

Houck, J.C., Sharma, V.K., and Cheng, R.F. (1973). *Nature New Biol. 246*: 111-113.

Houck, J.C., Weil, R.L., and Sharma, V.K. (1972). *Nature New Biol. 240*: 210-211.

Jainchill, J.L. and Todaro, G.J. (1970). *Exp. Cell Res. 59*: 137-146.

Kolodny, G.M. (1973). *J. Mol. Biol. 78*: 197-210.

Kruse, P.F., Jr. and Miedema, E. (1965). *J. Cell Biol. 27*: 273-279.

Kruse, P.F., Jr., Whittle, W., and Miedema, E. (1969). *J. Cell Biol. 42*: 113-121.

Laurence, E.B. (1973).*Natl. Cancer Inst. Monogr. 38*: 37-45.

Lee, J.C.K. (1971). *Am. J. Pathol. 65*: 347-356.

Lee, K., Sun, S., and Miller, O.N. (1968). *Arch. Biochem. Biophys. 125*: 751-757.

Leong, G.F., Grisham, J.W., Hole, B.V., and Albright, M.L. (1964). *Cancer Res. 24*: 1496-1501.

Levi-Montalcini, R. (1966). *Harvey Lect. 60*: 217-259.

Levine, S., Pictet, R.L., and Rutter, W.J. (1973). *Nature New Biol. 246*: 49-52.

Lipkin, G. and Knecht, M.E. (1974). *Proc. Natl. Acad. Sci. USA 71*: 849-853.

Loewenstein, W.R. (1973). *Fed. Proc. 32:* 60-64.

Mauel, J. and Defendi, V. (1971). *Exp. Cell Res. 65*: 33-42.

Metcalf, D. (1971). *Adv. Cancer Res. 14*: 181-230.

Oey, J., Vogel, A., and Pollack, R. (1974). *Proc. Natl. Acad. Sci. USA 71*: 694-698.

Paul, D., Lipton, A., and Klinger, I. (1971). *Proc. Natl. Acad. Sci. USA 68*: 645-648.

Paul, D. and Walter, S. (1974). *Proc. Soc. Exp. Biol. Med. 145*: 456-460.

Pickart, L. and Thaler, M.M. (1973). *Nature New Biol. 243*: 85-87.

Pierson, R.W. Jr. and Temin, H. M. (1972). *J. Cell. Physiol. 79*: 319-330.

Ponten, J. (1971). *Spontaneous and Virus Induced Transformation in Cell Culture.* Springer-Verlag, New York. pp. 12-15.

Rutter, W.J., Pictet, R.L., and Morris, T.W. (1973). *Ann. Rev. Biochem. 42*: 601-646.

Sachs, L. (1974). In *Control of Proliferation in Animal Cells*, B. Clarkson and R. Baserga (Eds.). Cold Spring Harbor Laboratory, pp. 915-925.

Scher, C.D., Stathakos, D., and Antoniades, H.N. (1974). *Nature 247*: 279-281.

Schnebli, H.P. and Haemmerli, G. (1974). *Nature 248*: 150-151.

Shodell, M. and Isselbacher, K. (1973). *Nature New Biol. 243*: 83-85.

Short, J., Armstrong, N.D., Zemel, R., and Lieverman, I. (1973). *Biochem. Biophys. Res. Comm. 50*: 430-437.

Short, J., Brown, R.F., Husakova, A., Gilbertson, J.R., Zemel, R., and Lieberman, I. (1972). *J. Biol. Chem. 247*: 1757-1766.

Short, J., Armstrong, N.B., Kolitsky, M.A., Mitchel, R.A., Zemel, R., and Lieberman, I. (1974). In *Control of Proliferation in Animal Cells*, B. Clarkson and R. Baserga (Eds.). Cold Spring Harbor Laboratory, pp. 37-48.

Simard, A., Corneille, L., Deschamps, Y., and Verly, W.E. (1974). *Proc. Natl. Acad. Sci. USA 71*: 1763-1766.

Stoker, M.G.P. (1973). *Nature 246*: 200-203.

Stoker, M.G.P. and Rubin H. (1967). *Nature 215*: 171-172.

Till, J.E., Messner, H.A., Price, G.B., Aye, M.T., and McCulloch, E.A., (1974). In *Control of Proliferation in Animal Cells*, B. Clarkson and R. Baserga (Eds.). Cold Spring Harbor Laboratory, pp. 907-913.

Vaheri, A., Ruoslahti, E., Hovi, T., and Nordling, S.J. (1973). *J. Cell. Physiol. 81*: 355-364.

Waymouth, C. (1965). In *Cells and Tissues in Culture, Vol. 1* E.N. Willmer (Ed.). Academic Press, New York, pp. 99-142.

Westermark, G. (1973). *Int. J. Cancer 12*: 438-451.

Wolstenholme, G.E.W. and Knight, J. (Eds.). *Homeostatic Regulators*. A Ciba Foundation Symposium. Churchill, London 1969, passim.

Yeh, J. and Fisher, H.W. (1969). *J. Cell Biol. 40*: 382-388.

ELEVEN

G_0 VERSUS G_1 CELLS

BIOLOGICAL DIFFERENCES

Promissio boni viri. . . . . . . It is now time to make good the promise made a few chapters ago of providing evidence that G_0 cells are different from G_1 cells. A glance at Figure 1.3 would, indeed suggest that the G_0 state is nothing else but a very long G_1. The question can be posed in a very simple way: either G_0 and G_1 cells cannot be distinguished from one another or they can be distinguished on the basis of some structural or functional difference. In the former case the G_0 state would not exist (except as a flatus vocis), but in the latter case that economy of language that is the hallmark of scientific endeavor would indicate the usefulness of designating certain cells as G_0 cells rather than cells in a very long G_1 state.

The concept of G_0 cells was introduced in 1963 by Lajtha to designate quiescent cells that do not synthesize DNA nor divide but that can be stimulated to do so by the application of an appropriate stimulus. It referred, therefore, mostly to cells like hepatocytes, cells of the renal tubules, salivary gland cells, and similar other cells of the adult animal, which in physiological conditions do not synthesize DNA nor undergo mitosis but can be induced to do so by appropriate stimuli. The concept of G_0

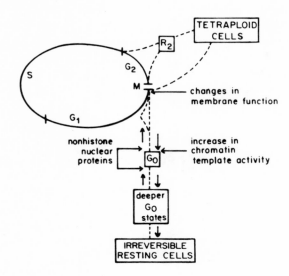

FIGURE 11-1   The perils of a cell. Continuously dividing cells
(lining epithelium of the crypts of the small intestine, exponentially
growing cells in culture) are cells that go around the cycle, from
one mitosis (M) to the next through G_1, S, and G_2. They can
leave the cycle either from G_2 or immediately after mitosis. Cells
leaving the cycle in G_2 can return to the cycle by reentering it
before (epidermal cells of mouse skin) or after M (tetraploid
hepatocytes). In the latter case, the tetraploid cell goes once around
the cycle and divides into two tetraploid cells. Cells leaving the
cycle after M go into a brief G_1, then into G_0 (certain density inhibited cells, uterine cells in the castrated animal, and so forth). The
cell can return from G_0 to G_1 (a step characterized by a prompt increase in chromatin template activity) or it can go into a deeper G_0
state (lymphocytes, cells left confluent for long periods of time).
Cells can return to the cycle even from this deeper G_0 state.
However, in some instances, they go into an irreversible state of
quiescence, which they do not leave except to die (polymorphonuclear
leukocytes, keratinizing cells of the epidermis).

cells has been opposed for a number of years by several investigators who feel that the term G_0 simply reflects an artificial division and that G_0 cells are simply cells with a very long G_1, which can be shortened under certain specific conditions. The argument goes that since the length of the S phase also varies greatly in the same type of cell and can be shortened by an appropriate stimulus, (for instance, the length of the S phase of mammary gland cells can be shortened by the administration of estrogens), the creation of a G_0 state would in turn, justify the creation of subclasses of S phase. In more recent years, however, evidence has been accumulating that G_0 cells can actually be distinguished on a functional basis from cells with a long G_1 and the general consensus nowadays is that G_0 cells do exist as separate entities (Epifanova and Terskikh 1969, Sander and Pardee 1972, Rovera and Baserga 1973, Smets 1973, Baserga et al. 1973). The task for the present chapter is to marshall the evidence accumulated thus far that favors such separation.

One direct approach to the problem is to investigate biological differences between continuously dividing cells (ie., epithelial cells lining the crypts of the small intestine, cells of the germinal centers of the lymph nodes, cells of the basal layer of the epidermis) and the putative G_0 cells mentioned above, (ie., hepatocytes, renal cells, and salivary gland cells). In fact, the first timid suggestion that G_0 cells could be distinguished on a functional basis from G_1 cells came in a rather round-about way when Becker and Broome (1967) found that L-asparaginase, while inhibiting mitotic response after partial hepatectomy, had no effect on mitotic activity of the gut or lymphoid tissue. These two classes of cells could also be differentiated on the basis of their response to the toxic effect of hydroxyurea. This drug inhibits DNA replication in both continuously dividing cells and in putative G_0 cells stimulated to synthesize DNA by an appropriate stimulus. However, after a single injection of hydroxyurea, continuously dividing cells in S phase disintegrate and die, whereas stimulated G_0 cells in S phase recover from the inhibition, complete DNA replication, and survive without any apparent damage (Farber and Baserga 1969).

CELL KINETICS

As we just mentioned, the anti-G_0 forces feel that a G_0 state is nothing else but a long G_1 peculiar to some kinds of cells. In fact, by comparing the length of the prereplicative phase of quiescent cells stimulated to proliferate with the length of G_1 in continuously dividing cells, it would seem that G_0 cells are cells like all others, but with a somewhat longer G_1, and that the length of G_1 is simply a characteristic of each cell type. However, some experiments in which putative G_0 cells have been repeatedly stimulated to proliferate indicate that the same cell type may display the kinetics of a G_0 or a G_1 cell.

In the isoproterenol-stimulated salivary glands of mice the length of the prereplicative phase, as we have already seen, is 20 hours. However, if a second injection of isoproterenol is given 48 hours after the first (at which time the salivary gland cells are again totally quiescent), the prereplicative phase is shortened to 14 hours (Novi and Baserga 1972). A similar situation has been described in human lymphocytes stimulated and subsequently restimulated with phytohemagglutinin (Younkin 1972). In fact, phytohemagglutinin-stimulated lymphocytes (at variance with the isoproterenol-stimulated salivary glands) go through more than one division cycle. The interval between the application of the stimulus and the onset of DNA synthesis is between 48 and 72 hours, but the first postmitotic G_1 period is very short, virtually nonexistent (Sören 1973).

Even better is the system described by Choie and Richter (1973). The length of the prereplicative phase in tubular epithelial cells of rat kidney stimulated to proliferate by a single injection of lead (0.05 mg/g body weight) is 20 hours. A second injection 48 hours after the first causes a second wave of DNA synthesis within 6 hours.

It is then possible to shorten, in the same cells, the interval between quiescence and the onset of DNA synthesis, which would indicate two different states of biochemical preparedness.

This situation is true also for cells in culture. For instance Sander and Pardee (1972) studied Chinese hamster ovary cells in culture, synchronized in two different ways. In some experiments the cells were detached from coverslips while in mitosis, and their behavior was followed directly as they passed from mitosis to G_1, S, and G_2 In other experiments the cells were arrested in a stationary phase by the isoleucine-deficiency technique of Ley and Tobey (1970). Sander and Pardee (1972) observed that the uptake of 2-amino-isobutyric acid by CHO cells doubled within 30 minutes after the cells detached from coverslips at mitosis had entered the G_1 period. Thereafter, the transport activity for 2-amino-isobutyric acid remained constant throughout the cell cycle, falling again at mitosis. However, when the same cells were arrested by isoleucine deprivation and the cell cycle traverse was initiated again by adding the missing amino acid, the uptake of 2-aminoisobutyric acid did not increase for at least 3 hours after the addition of isoleucine, then it doubled and remained elevated as in late G_1, S, or G_2 of mitotically detached cells. There was, therefore, a difference of 2½ hours in the time required for the doubling of the transport rate of 2-aminoisobutyric acid between the cells entering G_1 directly from mitosis and cells entering G_1 after isoleucine deprivation. Interestingly enough, the time required by isoleucine-synchronized CHO cells to complete G_1 and begin DNA synthesis was from 2 to 3 hours longer than for cells synchronized by mitotic selection. Sander and Pardee (1972) felt that the isoleucine-blocked cells were in a different state, ie., G_0, than growing cells right after mitosis, ie., in early G_1, and that this difference was evidenced both by the different lengths of the prereplicative phase and by the time differences in the membrane transport changes.

We shall return to membrane changes in G_0 and G_1 cells in this same chapter, but, at this point, we should like to mention the possibility that, let alone G_0, different levels of G_0 may actually exist. When WI-38 human diploid fibroblasts are left to grow in the medium originally used for plating, they form confluent monolayers and become quiescent by the day 5. If the old medium is replaced by fresh medium and serum, cell proliferation is stimu-

lated anew, as we have already seen in chapter 5. However, the
length of the prereplicative phase increases with the time of quiescence.
Cells stimulated on day 5 reach DNA synthesis in 8 hours; cells
stimulated on day 9 in 14 hours and, finally, cells stimulated on
the day 18 have a prereplicative phase of 20 hours (Augenlicht
and Baserga 1974). Similar conclusions were reached by Gunther
et al. (1974) with lectin-stimulated lymphocytes. The kinetics of
cellular commitment in concanavalin A-stimulated lymphocytes
seem to indicate that individual lymphocytes are in different G_0
states. Does the G_0 state consist then, like Dante's Inferno, of
different levels of depth?

    Indeed, the length of the prereplicative phase in cells of
the cultured rabbit lens, triggered into DNA synthesis by a nutritional change, varies with the position of the cell in the lens itself
(Harding et al. 1968). This is an example of space-conditioned
level of G_0, but there are also examples of time-dependent levels
of G_0. Apart from the finding on WI-38 cells mentioned above, it
is well established that there is a lengthening of the prereplicative
phase in stimulated G_0 cells of old animals. For instance, after
partial hepatectomy hepatocytes of older rats take a longer time
to enter DNA synthesis than those of younger animals (Bucher
1963). Similar results have been reported in the isoproterenol-
stimulated salivary gland (Adelman et al. 1972), almost suggesting
that aging is accompanied by a deeper G_0 state. But this is part of
another story.

DIFFERENCES IN CONSTITUENT PROTEINS

    Kinetic considerations therefore suggest some differences
between bona fide G_1 and putative G_0 cells. Another approach to
the problem of separating G_0 from G_1 cells is to investigate possible
biochemical differences between growing and stationary cells in culture. Thus, in continuously dividing HeLa cells the repair enzyme
DNA polymerase has a constant activity throughout the cell cycle
from early G_1 to mitosis (Friedman 1970). However, in stationary

cells DNA polymerase activity is much lower than in growing cells
(Adams et al. 1965). In hamster fibroblasts in culture Becker et al.
(1971) found that stationary cells (which they classified as G_0
cells) had a ribosome complement that was only 70% of the ribosome
complement of G_1 cells. Differences have also been found in certain soluble cellular proteins that have the property of binding
tightly to DNA cellulose columns. Thus, whereas most DNA-binding
proteins are synthesized essentially at the same rate throughout the
cell cycle of mouse fibroblasts (except for histones that are synthesized
only during the S phase), stationary cells synthesize certain DNA
binding proteins that are not synthesized during the cell cycle of
growing cells (Fox and Pardee 1971). Similar conclusions were
reached by Becker and Stanners (1972) who showed that the gel
electrophoretic profiles of nonhistone chromosomal proteins of
L-mouse fibroblasts are substantially similar in the various phases
of the cell cycle, from early G_1 to mitosis. However, when the same
cells were in stationary phase, the gel electrophoretic profile of nonhistone chromosomal proteins showed specific and reproducible
differences in comparison to cycling cells.

Finally, in human fibroblasts quiescent for 3 or more
weeks there is a 30% loss in the amount of total cellular proteins
(Dell'Orco et al. 1973).

TRANSFORMED AND UNTRANSFORMED CELLS

These findings therefore indicate that there are differences in the protein complement of G_1 cells and of stationary cells.
However, it would be a mistake to identify and equate stationary
cells with G_0 cells. On the contrary, it is important to realize that
cells in culture may arrest either in G_1 of G_0. An evident demonstration of this possibility has been furnished by the experiments
of Sander and Pardee (1972) described above, which indicate that
the same type of cell may arrest either in G_1 or in G_0, from which
phase it may take a longer time to again reach the DNA synthesis
phase. Furthermore, it is possible that some cell lines in culture

may ordinarily arrest in G_1, while other cells may arrest in the G_0 state. This possibility is clearly illustrated by differences in the stationary phase of WI-38 human diploid fibroblasts on one side and 3T6 mouse fibroblasts or SV-40 transformed human fibroblasts (2RA) on the other. For instance, the stimulation of confluent monolayers of quiescent diploid WI-38 cells requires the addition of fresh serum. Change of medium, without addition of fresh serum (or addition of insufficient amounts of serum), does not cause stimulation. On the contrary, both 2RA fibroblasts and 3T6 cells, which are rightly considered as transformed cells (Todaro 1972), respond promptly with a marked stimulation of cell proliferation to a simple replacement of the conditioned medium by fresh medium, even without serum (Baserga et al. 1973). In addition, the interval between the application of the stimulus and the onset of DNA synthesis is also shorter in 3T6 mouse fibroblasts and in SV-40 transformed human fibroblasts than in WI-38 cells. The difference is about 3 hours, as if that particular length of time, very similar to the one reported by Sander and Pardee (1972) for CHO cells, were required for the transition from the G_0 state to the G_1 phase. Confirming the findings of Sander and Pardee (1972), Costlow and Baserga (1973) observed that when quiescent WI-38 human diploid fibroblasts are stimulated to proliferate by a change of medium and fresh serum, there is no increase in the uptake of cycloleucine or 2-deoxyglucose until 3 hours after stimulation. The transport rate of these two compounds then roughly doubles and remains constant throughout the length of the cell cycle. On the contrary, in cells like 3T6 and 2RA the uptake of low molecular weight compounds increases immediately after stimulation. The findings of Sander and Pardee (1972) and Costlow and Baserga (1973) may explain a discrepancy that has puzzled investigators for a number of years. Thus, it has been known for a long time that when aneuploid stationary cells in culture are stimulated by nutritional changes, there is a prompt increase in the uptake of low molecular weight compounds such as amino acids and nucleosides (see chapter 9). This finding, in aneuploid cells like 3T3, 3T6, and so on, is so common that (*e pluribus unum*) the several observations inevitably culminated in a theory, the theory of the *pleiotypic response* (Hershko et al. 1971). On the other hand, in quiescent diploid fibroblasts stimulated by a change of medium, it was found that in the 2 hours after stimulation the uptake of aminoacid actually decreased (Wiebel and Baserga 1969). A similar delay of 2 hours in the increased transport of uridine occurs in the estrogen-stimulated uterus (Billing et al. 1969). The difference may be explained by supposing that confluent diploid fibroblasts are in G_0, whereas cells like 3T6, 2RA, and so on, are arrested, except under certain specific conditions, in early G_1.

CHROMATIN TEMPLATE ACTIVITY

If it is true that WI-38 cells are arrested in G_0 while 2RA and 3T6 cells are arrested in G_1, then it should be possible to distinguish these two kinds of cells on the basis of chromatin template activity after stimulation. It has been shown in chapter 6 that it is a characteristic of putative G_0 cells to respond with an increase in chromatin template activity to a stimulus to proliferate. This increase, about 50%-70% above control values, seems to be characteristic of all kinds of G_0 cells from the estrogen stimulated uterus to the isoproterenol stimulated salivary gland. On the other hand, continuously dividing cells behave in a different way. Johnson and Holland (1965) and Farber et al. (1972), have shown that during mitosis there is a marked decrease in chromatin template activity. However, the difference is almost fourfold (reflecting the absence of RNA synthesis in the intact mitotic cell), and once the cell has entered the G_1 period, chromatin template activity remains essentially the same throughout the cycle. As mentioned above, quiescent confluent monolayers of WI-38 human diploid fibroblasts show an increase in chromatin template activity within 1 hour after they are stimulated by a change of medium. However, density inhibited SV-40 transformed WI-38 human fibroblasts (2RA), do not show any increase in chromatin template activity when stimulated to proliferate by an appropriate nutritional change (Costlow and Baserga 1973). Similarly, 3T6 cells do not show any change in chromatin tem-

plate activity when stimulated to proliferate after reaching the
stationary phase (Rovera and Baserga 1973). Another prediction
of this model is that chromatin template activity (a) should not
increase in WI-38 cells stimulated on day 5 after plating, when they
are still in G_1 (see above); (b) should increase in WI-38 stimulated
between days 7 and 9 after plating, when they have entered G_0 ; and
(c) should also increase, but with a delay, in cells stimulated on day
18 after plating, that have a prolonged prereplicative phase. This
prediction was borne out precisely as stated above by Augenlicht
and Baserga (1974), and similar results were obtained by Smets
(1973) with 3T3 cells left quiescent for different lengths of time.

MECHANISM OF G_0 TRANSITION

It seems, therefore, that one may be justified in separating
G_0 from G_1 cells in the basis of several parameters which include:
(a) time differences in the length of the prereplicative phase; (b)
ability to respond with an increase in cell proliferation to nutritional changes; (c) differences in protein complement; (d) time
differences in changes occurring in membrane functions; and (e)
differences in the levels of chromatin template activity. From
the data presented above, it would seem that the same type of
cell may arrest in either G_0 or G_1 but there are some cell lines that
find it more difficult to enter G_0 than others. In this connection
it seems likely that some minor revisions may be necessary in de-
scribing the growth patterns of cells in culture. It has been customary
to say that cells go through an exponential phase of growth after
which they reach a stationary phase during which they are density
inhibited. It becomes increasingly clear that the stationary phase
can consist of at least two different phases, ie., a G_1 and a G_0
phase. This concept, by the way, is the same as the one first
introduced by Temin (1971) in his experiments with chick embryo
fibroblasts in which he used the term G_{1b} instead of G_0 .

A few words should be said about possible mechanisms
responsible for the G_0 transition. The data of Engelhardt on Vero

cells in stationary phases are relevant here. When Vero cells reach a stationary phase, the amount of proteins synthesized is markedly depressed, a phenomenon common also to other cell lines (Levine et al. 1965). Engelhardt (1971) showed that the inhibition of protein synthesis is accompanied by the appearance of an inhibitory agent that blocks protein synthesis in cell-free amino acid incorporating systems isolated from these cells. The inhibitory agent, which has been partially purified, is obtained by freezing and thawing cytoplasmic extracts of cells which have been in the stationary phase of the growth cycle for 1 to 2 days. If the cells are in the stationary phase for longer than 2 days, the inhibitor of protein synthesis is found free in the cytoplasm even before the freezing and thawing step. The studies of Engelhardt (1971) could be explained by assuming that at first the growing Vero cells enter a phase of G_1, during which an inhibitor makes its appearance but is tightly bound to the polyribosomes, and then finally step into the G_0 phase recognizable by the appearance of the inhibitory agent in the soluble fraction of the cell. Another possible mechanism is based on the above mentioned observations that there are differences in the nonhistone chromosomal proteins of growing and stationary cells (see also chapter 7). Allfrey et al. (1975) have found that stimulation of lymphocytes with concanavalin A causes a dramatic migration of preexisting nonhistone chromosomal proteins from the cytoplasm to nuclear chromatin. A similar migration of presynthesized nuclear proteins from HeLa cells has been described in chick nuclei when chick erythrocytes are fused with HeLa cells (Appels et al. 1974). Along the same lines, while there is no appreciable increase in the amount of nuclear proteins in confluent monolayers of WI-38 cells stimulated to proliferate by a change of medium, the nuclear content of proteins increases 40% in WI-38 cells stimulated to proliferate by trypsinization and re seeding at lower densities (Maizel et al. 1975). It should be noted that trypsinization of WI-38 cells causes a 30%-40% loss of nonhistone chromosomal proteins from the nucleus and an increase in the length of the prereplicative phase from 12 to 20 hours. These experiments would suggest that cells in deep G_0 (such as lymphocytes, chick erythrocytes, and trypsinized WI-38 fibroblasts) may have lost some nonhistone chromosomal proteins that have to be restored to the nucleus before the regular G_0 can begin. An analogous conclusion was reached by Gordon and Cohn (1971) when they observed that the activation of chick red cell nuclei fused with melanocytes took longer than 10 hours, while 80% of the macrophage nuclei initiated DNA synthesis in the 3-7 hour period after fusion. They felt that "the lag before DNA synthesis may reflect the heterochromatin content of each nucleus."

A third possible mechanism responsible for sending a cell into the Nirvana of G_0 is a decrease in the synthesis of ribosomal RNA. A decrease in ribosomal RNA synthesis when cells switched from exponential growth to stationary phase has been described in chick fibroblasts (Emerson 1971; Weber 1972) and in CVI cells (Rovera et al. 1975). In all these instances the synthesis of heterogeneous nuclear RNA is only slightly affected or not at all. However, it would seem, at first blush, that the decreased synthesis of ribosomal RNA in stationary cells is the effect, rather than the cause, of the G_0 transition.

In any case it seems safe to conclude from these data that G_0 and G_1 cells can be distinguished from each other on the basis of different biochemical features and that the G_0 state is usually obtained by confluent cells only after they have been in a stationary phase for some period of time. Whether the neoplastic transformation may involve decreased ability of some cells to enter the G_0 phase will be discussed in chapter 13.

For the moment, we shall limit ourselves to modifying Figure 1-3 and to give a new, more elaborate diagram of the vicissitudes of a cell, which we could entitle either Figure 11-1, or the *Perils of a Cell*. Since the explanation of Figure 11-1 is given in the legend, it will not be repeated here. The reader will forgive me for breaking the rule of William of Occam that *Entia non sunt multiplicanda praeter necessitatem*. However, like the characters besieging the writer in one of Pirandello's novels, many types of cells clamored for recognition from the pages of literature. And each of them wanted a name.

REFERENCES

Adams, R.L.P., Abrams, R., and Lieberman, I. (1965). *Nature 206*: 512-513.

Adelman, R.C., Stein, G., Roth, G.S., and Englander, D. (1972). *Mech. Age Dev. 1*: 49-59.

Allfrey, V.G., Inoue, A., Johnson, E.M., and Karn, J. (1975). In *The Structure and Function of Chromatin*. Ciba Foundation Symposium, London, pp. 199-219.

Appels, R., Bolund, L., Goto, S., and Ringertz, N.R. (1974). *Exp. Cell Res. 85*: 182-190.

Augenlicht, L. and Baserga, R. (1974). *Exp. Cell Res. 89*: 255-262.

Baserga, R., Costlow, M., and Rovera, G. (1973). *Fed. Proc. 32*: 2115-2118.

Becker, F.F. and Broome, J.D. (1967). *Science 156*: 1602-1603.

Becker, H. and Stanners, C.P. (1972). *J. Cell. Physiol. 80*: 51-61.

Becker, H., Stanners, C.P., and Kudlow, J.E. (1971). *J. Cell. Physiol. 77*: 43-50.

Billing, R.J., Barbiroli, B., and Smellie, R.M.S. (1969). *Biochim. Biophys. Acta 190*: 52-59.

Bucher, N.L.R. (1963). *Int. Rev. Cytol. 15*: 245-300.

Choie, D.D. and Richter, G.W. (1973). *Proc. Soc. Exp. Biol. Med. 142*: 446-449.

Costlow, M. and Baserga, R. (1973). *J. Cell. Physiol. 82*: 411-420.

Dell'Orco, R.T., Mertens, J.G., and Kruse, P.F. Jr. (1973). *Exp. Cell Res. 77*: 356-360.

Emerson, C.P., Jr. (1971). *Nature New Biol. 232*: 101-106.

Engelhardt, D.L. (1971). *J. Cell. Physiol. 78*: 333-343.

Epifanova, O.I. and Terskikh, V.V. (1969). *Cell Tissue Kinet. 2*: 75-93.

Farber, E. and Baserga, R. (1969). *Cancer Res. 29*: 136-139.

Farber, J., Stein, G., and Baserga, R. (1972). *Biochem. Biophys. Res. Comm. 47*: 790-797.

Fox, T.O. and Pardee, A.B. (1971). *Biol. Chem. 246*: 6159-6165.

Friedman, D.L. (1970). *Biochem. Biophys. Res. Comm. 39*: 100-109.

Gordon, S. and Cohn, Z. (1971). *J. Exp. Med. 133*: 321-338.

Gunther, G.R., Wang, J.L., and Edelman, G.M. (1974). *J. Cell. Biol. 62*: 366-377.

Harding, C.V., Wilson, W.L., Wilson, J.R., Reddan, J.R., and Reddy, V.N. (1968). *J. Cell. Physiol. 72*: 213-220.

Hershko, A., Mamont, P. Shields, R., and Tomkins, G.M. (1971). *Nature New Biol. 232*: 206-211.

Johnson, T.C. and Holland, J.J. (1965). *J. Cell. Biol. 27*: 565-574.

Lajtha, L.G. (1962). *Postgrad. Med. J. 38:* 41-47.

Levine, E.M., Becker, Y., Boone, C.W., and Eagle, H. (1965). *Proc. Natl. Acad. Sci. USA 53*: 350-356.

Ley, K.D. and Tobey, R.A. (1970). *J. Cell. Biol. 47*: 453-459.

Maizel, A., Nicolini, C., and Baserga, R. (1975). *J. Cell. Physiol. 86*: 71-82.

Novi, A.M. and Baserga, R. (1972). *Lab. Invest. 26*: 540-547.

Rovera, G. and Baserga, R. (1973). *Exp. Cell Res. 78*: 118-126.

Rovera, G., Metha, S. and Maul, G. (1975). *Exp. Cell Res. 89*: 295-305.

Smets, L.A. (1973). *Exp. Cell Res. 79*: 239-243.

Sören, L. (1973). *Exp. Cell Res. 78*: 231-233.

Temin, H.M. (1971). *J. Cell. Physiol. 78*: 161-170.

Todaro, G. (1972). *Nature New Biol. 240*: 157-160.

Weber, M.J. (1972). *Nature New Biol. 235*: 58-61.

Wiebel, F. and Baserga, R. (1969). *J. Cell Physiol. 74*: 191-202.

Younkin, L.H. (1972). *Exp. Cell Res. 75*: 1-10.

TWELVE

HYPERTROPHY AND HYPERPLASIA

CELL NUMBER AND SIZE

Division of cells does not necessarily mean multiplication. We have seen in previous chapters that when the rate of cell loss equals the rate of production of new cells, the number of cells in the population remains constant. It is only when the rate of production of new cells exceeds the rate of cell loss that a cell population increases, that is, grows. However, there is another mechanism through which a tissue or an organ may grow and that is by increasing the size of cells. These two mechanisms of growth (increase in cell number and increase in cell size) are so basic that they are found even in unicellular organisms. Thus, a single bacterium will produce a colony visible to the naked eye through the continuous multiplcation of bacterial cells. At the opposite end of the spectrum is the unicellular alga, *Acetabularia*, which has been an extremely useful laboratory tool for the study of differentiation (for a discussion see the delightful book *Nucleus and Cytoplasm* by Harris 1968). Acetabularia grows from a small zygote into a plant 3-5 cm long which contains a single nucleus located in the tip of one of the rhizoids at the base of its stalk. Acetabularia, that is, grows exclusively by increasing its size.

These same basic mechanisms extend to multicellular organisms, but in this case tissues or organs can use a variation of the increase in cell size, which is the increase in the amount of intercellular substance. Thus, bone or connective tissue can increase in size by increasing the amount of intercellular substances, while the size and number of cells remain unchanged. However, since the intercellular substance is secreted by cells and can therefore be considered an extension of the cell cytoplasm, an increase in intercellular substance can be interpreted as a simple variation of the increase in cell size. With this qualification in mind it is easy to see that tissues or organs of multicellular organisms also follow the two basic mechanisms described above and can grow either by increasing the number or the size of the cells. As an illustration of these two mechanisms we may take the last vestigial symbols of male chauvinism, that is the deer's antlers and the cock's comb. The deer's antlers grow every spring at a fantastic speed because of the continuous and extremely rapid proliferation of progenitor cells at the base of the antlers. On the other hand, the cock's comb grows to its gallant size by increasing the size of cells and especially the amount of intercellular substance which, in the case of the cock's comb, is mostly hyaluronic acid and its derivatives (Szirmai 1962).

Abnormal growth can also be due to either of these two mechanisms, and this has been recognized for many decades by pathologists who have distinguished hyperplasia (increase in the number of cells) from hypertrophy (increase in the size of the cells). For instance, hyperplasia of the parathyroid glands is a condition in which the number of parathyroid cells is increased. On the other hand, cardiac hypertrophy (ie., enlargement of the heart) has always been considered a condition in which the size, but not the number of myocardial cells, is considerably increased. The two processes have always been kept sharply separated even at a subcellular level, with hyperplasia considered mainly a nuclear process (the increased number of cells being due to mitoses) and hypertrophy an exclusively cytoplasmic alteration. Thus, it is clearly stated in a textbook of pathology that in hypertrophy a tissue ". . .can grow only by increasing the cytoplasmic mass of individual cells" (Robbins 1962).

Unfortunately, cells do not read our textbooks, and in recent years a number of observations have raised serious doubts about the definition of hypertrophy as an exclusively cytoplasmic process, as well as to the sharp distinction between hypertrophy and hyperplasia.

A milestone in this respect was the observation of Sandritter and Scomazzoni (1964) that the DNA content of hypertrophic myocardial cells was higher than the DNA content of normal myocardial cells. These authors showed that 95% of the myocardial nuclei from adult hearts of normal weight were tetraploid (4 C amount of DNA). In severely hypertrophic hearts as many as 82% of the myocardial nuclei were octoploid (8 C), while the remainder had 16 C and even 32 C amounts of DNA. It is interesting that myocardial nuclei from normal adult hearts are already tetraploid. In children below 3 years of age, 85% of the myocardial nuclei are diploid and only 15% are tetraploid (Fischer et al. 1970). Polyploidization occurs between 3 and 8 years of age, a phenomenon similar to what occurs in the liver of experimental animals, as will be detailed below. The findings of Sandritter and coworkers on human hearts have been confirmed by Eisenstein and Wied (1970), and indicate that although the myocardial fibers may increase notably in size during the hypertrophic process the nucleus is not a passive passenger but, on the contrary, it undergoes reduplication of DNA, even several times, reaching a size that is apparently commensurate with the size of the whole cell. To complicate matters further, together with the cytoplasmic enlargement and the increased amount of DNA per nucleus, there is, in hypertrophic hearts, an increase in the number of cells, both connective tissue cells and myocardial cells (Sandritter and Adler 1971). The prototype of hypertrophy, cardiac enlargement, has now become a perfect example of how closely interrelated are hyperplasia and hypertrophy, cytoplasmic and nuclear events.

EXPERIMENTAL HYPERTROPHY

A similar situation can be reproduced experimentally. The reader is by now familiar with the isoproterenol-stimulated mouse salivary gland in which a single injection of isoproterenol causes, after a lag period of about 20 hours, a marked stimulation of DNA synthesis in the acinar cells of the parotid and submaxillary glands, followed by a wave of mitoses. According to the definition given, this is a typical example of hyperplasia. However, if isoproterenol is injected, not just once but daily for several days, the salivary glands keep increasing in size and dry weight, although mitoses are no longer detectable (Schneyer et al. 1967). Let us take as an example the parotid glands of mice given repeated injections of isoproterenol (Novi and Baserga 1971). The amount of DNA per nucleus in a normal parotid gland is 9.9×10^{-12} g. After four injections of isoproterenol, the DNA content per nucleus increases to an average of 18.4×10^{-12} g and after 10 injections of isoproterenol, to an average of 27.9×10^{-12} g per nucleus. The mitotic index which is 45 per 1,000 cells 24 hours after a single injection of isoproterenol, decreases to 25 per 1000 after 4 days of treatment and to 0 after 10 days of treatment. Radley (1968) showed that this is due to an increase in the number of polyploid cells. Thus, the increase in size and dry weight of the salivary glands after repeated injections of isoproterenol is not due to cell division but is accompanied by a marked increase in the amount of DNA per nucleus.

It would therefore seem that contrary to tradition hypertrophy is not a pure cytoplasmic event, but, on the contrary, is accompanied in man and in experimental animals by a considerable increase in the amount of DNA per nucleus. If this is correct, then hypertrophy and hyperplasia are not totally different processes but simply segments of different lengths of the same story. In fact, these findings raise the possibility that hypertrophy and hyperplasia may share, to a large extent, common biochemical events, at least up to the completion of DNA synthesis, that is, at the S/G_2 boundary. In other words, at least in some instances, the hypertrophic cell could simply be considered a G_2 blocked cell, a phenomenon that is known to happen under physiological conditions in a number of tissues. Tetraploid cells (with G_2 content of diploid cell's DNA) are quite common in certain tissues, as for instance in liver and in the central nervous system. An excellent demonstration of the interrelationship of cell size, nuclear ploidy, and cell number can be found in the studies of Fukuda and Sibatani (1953) in the growing rat liver. The data of Fukada and Sibatani (1953) are summarized in Table 12.1, from which it can be seen that: (a) there is a remarkable increase in the number of liver cells between 10 and 41 days after birth; (b) the amount of DNA per nucleus doubles between 21 and 41 days; and (c) the cell size (mass) increases sharply between 21 and 41 days (at the same time as the DNA content of nuclei) and more slowly thereafter. The rat liver in its postnatal growth therefore offers a clear example of how hyperplasia and hypertrophy can both contribute to the growth of an organ and of how an increase in cell size is correlated to an increase in the amount of DNA per nucleus.

The polyploidization of rat liver nuclei is, at least in part, controlled by sexual hormones (Swartz et al. 1960), and it is, therefore, not surprising that very little hypertrophy occurs in the prenatal period. Thus, Lafarge and Frayssinet (1964) divide the development of rat liver into three phases: (a) from days 15 to 18 of fetal life, growth by hyperplasia without hypertrophy; (b) from day 19 of fetal life to postnatal day 3, a period of cellular rearrangement; and (c) from postnatal day 3, growth by hypertrophy and hyperplasia.

Table 12-1   **Postnatal Growth of Rat Liver**[a]

Age (days)	Liver wt. (g)	Cell number ($\times 10^{-6}$)	Amt. per average cell DNA (pg)	protein (pg)	Cell mass (ng)
10	0.30	168	5.9	175	1.79
21	0.98	445	5.1	273	2.20
41	5.7	1060	11.1	618	5.36
80	8.1	1270	11.4	924	6.37
182	12.0	1790	11.4	930	6.70

[a] Modified from Fukuda and Sibatani (1953).

Liver and heart are not the only tissues that contain tetraploid cells in physiological conditions. Purkinje cells in the cerebellar cortex of rat and man are also tetraploid (Novakova et al. 1970), and an increase in the amount of DNA per cell is also apparent during the growth of several other organs (Winick and Noble 1965). Finally, another beautiful illustration of the relationship between cell mass and amount of DNA per nucleus can be found in the erythrocytes of amphibians, reptiles, and birds (Allfrey et al. 1955).

MOLECULAR BASIS OF HYPERTROPHY

If a hypertrophic cell is just a G_2 blocked cell, how can one predict whether a diploid cell stimulated to grow will divide or will, instead, become a tetraploid cell? Following our usual criteria, it would be necessary to identify certain biochemical events that occur in cells stimulated to divide, but not in cells stimulated to grow in size or vice versa. Excluded from these events are those occurring in G_2 and mitosis which represent the end point and, by definition, distinguish one kind of cell from another. What we are asking ourselves is whether it is possible to distinguish a cell destined to divide from a cell destined to stop in G_2 while they are both in the prereplicative phase preceding the onset of DNA synthesis or in the S phase itself. However, at the present moment, little information is available that may allow us to distinguish the prereplicative phase and the S phase of the cell stimulated to divide from those of the cell stimulated to grow in size. If DNA synthesis occurs in both instances, it is reasonable to assume that the various events preceding the onset of DNA synthesis in cells stimulated to divide, which we have been studying in previous chapters, will also occur in cells stimulated to grow in size. This is, in essence, what has been reported so far. However, a few timid suggestions have appeared that some differences may exist. These possible differences considered here are: (a) the nature of the very early events between the application of the stimulus and the activation of the chromatin

.template; (b) a difference in sensitivity to immunosuppressive agents; and (c) the requirement for ribosomal RNA synthesis.

GROWTH INDUCED BY SEX HORMONES

The estrogen-stimulated uterus is an example of a tissue in which cells are stimulated both to divide and to grow in size. In the uterine epithelium, the growth fraction increases from 8.3% in the ovariectomized mouse to 27.9% in estrogen treated mice (Epifanova 1971). However, together with this stimulation of cell proliferation there is also a considerable increase in the size of uterine cells (Hamilton 1968). According to Hamilton's data, treatment of ovariectomized rats with 17β-estradiol causes an increase in wet weight of the uterus from 68 to 210 mg (an increase of 3.1-fold). The DNA in the uterus increases only 1.26-fold (from 0.98 mg to 1.24 mg), and two ratios that usually give an approximate indication of the relative size of the cells also increase after estrogen treatment. The RNA:DNA ratio increases 1.9-fold, from 0.43 to 0.82, and the protein:DNA ratio increases 3.7-fold, from 2.1 to 7.82. In other words, although both processes are present in the estrogen-stimulated uterus, there is more hypertrophy than hyperplasia. It is possible that the mechanisms and biochemical events occurring between the application of the stimulus and the onset of DNA synthesis, discussed in previous chapters, may not be applicable in their totality to the estrogen-stimulated uterus. The pioneer work of Jensen and his coworkers and of Gorsky and his collaborators (summarized in a recent review by Jensen and DeSombre 1973) has demonstrated that estrogens bind to a receptor complex in the cytoplasm and eventually reach the nucleus as a receptor-estrogen complex. This estrogen-receptor complex binds to the chromatin of the target organ but not to the chromatin of other nontarget tissues (Steggles et al. 1971). The nature of the binding of the receptor-estrogen (or progesterone) complex to the nuclear acceptor has been very lucidly reviewed by O'Malley and Means (1974), and although it is not yet clear whether the nuclear acceptor is an acidic or a basic protein (Puca et al. 1974), it seems

reasonable to assume that female steroid hormones interact, indirectly, with chromatin. Indeed, Mohla et al. (1972)
have shown that this estrogen-receptor complex, once bound to
chromatin, activates the chromatin and increases its template
activity. An analogous situation has been described in the proges-
terone-stimulated chick oviduct (O'Malley et al. 1970, Steggles et al.
1971) where hypertrophy is again more accentuated than hyperplasia. Here also, the progesterone-receptor complex binds directly
to chromatin and more specifically, to a nonhistone chromosomal
protein (Spelsberg et al. 1971). Therefore in the case of steroid
hormones, such as estrogens and progesterone one could postulate
that the increased chromatin template activity is directly caused
by the steroid-receptor complex and that the activation of chromatin does not involve the previous synthesis of a nonhistone
nuclear protein. More important, the earliest detectable hormonal
response in estrogen-stimulated uterus is an increase in RNA polymerase II activity, which is detectable within 10-15 minutes and
precedes the increase in chromatin template activity (Glasser et
al. 1972, and see also the review by O'Malley and Means 1974).

   It could be that while both hypertrophy and hyperplasia
share an increase in chromatin template activity, the events preceding this increase may be slightly different. It should be noted
at this point that the transcriptional activity of chromatin is increased even in those systems in which hypertrophy is predominant
and hyperplasia is minimal, as in rat adrenal glands stimulated by
ACTH (Alvarez and Lavender 1974).

                         IMMUNOSUPPRESSIVE AGENTS

   The possibility that immunosuppressive agents may be
able to distinguish between hypertrophy and hyperplasia is given
by two reports that have appeared in the literature. The first one
is the report of DeCosse and Gelfant (1968) who showed that G_2
cells can be triggered into mitosis by the administration of the immunosuppressive steroid hormone, cortisone. Even more signifi-

cant are the experiments of Malamud et al. (1972) who showed that azathioprine (at a dose of 40 mg/kg) inhibits cell proliferation but not hypertrophy in rat liver following partial hepatectomy. The liver cells increase considerably in size in azathioprine-treated partially hepatectomized rats, but do not divide, although G_2 cells do undergo mitosis. These experiments should be construed as suggesting that immunosuppressive agents on one side inhibit the flow of cells from G_0 to mitosis and, on the other side, trigger mitosis in G_2-blocked cells.

RNA

The role of ribosomal RNA in cell proliferation has already been discussed in previous chapters. A number of investigators have reported that the synthesis of rRNA is a requirement for cell growth (Tata 1968 and 1970, Becker et al. 1971, Baserga 1971, Johnson et al. 1974). However, Studzinski and Gierthy (1973) have shown that while the synthesis of ribosomal RNA is an essential prerequisite for cell division in diploid cells, aneuploid cells can undergo at least one mitotic division in the almost total absence of ribosomal RNA synthesis. When rRNA synthesis is inhibited by the aminonucleoside of puromycin, diploid fibroblasts stop dividing but continue to synthesize DNA. In addition, in the temperature-sensitive mutant described by Toniolo et al. (1973), in which 28S ribosomal RNA is not produced at the nonpermissive temperature, the mutant cells stop dividing after one mitosis, but then continue to increase in size, reaching monstrous proportions. In this particular case it seems that the lack of production of 28S ribosomal RNA causes an unbalanced growth, with continued DNA synthesis but without cell division. If these findings were to be confirmed in other models, they would suggest that ribosomal RNA synthesis is more necessary to mitosis than to the reduplication of DNA. However, as mentioned above these are extremely tentative conclusions based on a few recent experiments that require confirmation and further detailed investigations.

For the moment we shall simply conclude this chapter by reminding the reader again that the classical distinction between hypertrophy and hyperplasia is now somewhat obscured, and that many of the biochemical events occurring in cells stimulated to divide also occur in cells stimulated to grow in size. Such a conclusion would make hypertrophy and hyperplasia two essentially similar processes distinguished only by diverging end points. With these two examples of altered growth, the stage is properly set for studying the cancer cell, which is the best known example of abnormal growth and, at the same time, the most baffling and most difficult to explain.

References

Allfrey, V.G., Mirsky, A.E, and Stern, H. (1955). *Adv. Enzymol. 16*: 411-492.
Alvarez, M.R. and Lavender, K. (1974). *Exp. Cell Res. 83*: 1-8.
Baserga, R. (Ed.). The Cell Cycle and Cancer. Marcel Dekker, New York, 1971, passim.
Becker, H., Stanners, C.P., and Kudlow, J.E. (1971). *J. Cell Physiol. 77*: 43-50.
DeCosse, J.J. and Gelfant, S. (1968). *Science 162*: 698-699.
Eisenstein, R. and Wied, G.L. (1970). *Proc. Soc. Exp. Biol. Med. 134*: 176-179.
Epifanova, O.I. (1971). In *The Cell Cycle and Cancer,* R. Baserga (Ed.). Marcel Dekker, New York, pp. 145-190.
Fischer, B., Schulter, G., Adler, C.P., and Sandritter, W. (1970). *Beitr. Pathol. 141*: 238-260.
Fukuda, M. and Sibatani, A. (1953). *J. Biochem. 40*: 95-110.
Glasser, S.R., Chytil, F., and Spelsberg, T.C. (1972). *Biochem. J. 130*: 947-957.
Hamilton, T.H. (1968). *Science 161*: 649-661.
Harris, H. (1968). *Nucleus and Cytoplasm*. Clarendon Press, Oxford.
Jensen, E.V. and DeSombre, E.R. (1973). *Science 182*: 126-134.
Johnson, L.F., Abelson, H.T., Green, H., and Penman, S. (1974). *Cell 1*: 33-38.
Lafarge, C., and Frayssinet, C. (1964). *Bull. Soc. Chimie Biol. 46*: 1045-1057.
Malamud, D., Gonzalez, E.M., Chiu, H., and Malt, R.A. (1972). *Cancer Res. 32*: 1226-1229.
Mohla, S., DeSombre, E.R., and Jensen, E.V. (1972). *Biophys. Res. Comm. 46*: 661-667.

Novakova, V., Sandritter, W., and Schlueter, G. (1970). *Exp. Cell Res. 60*: 454-456.

Novi, A.M. and Baserga, R. (1971). *Am. J. Pathol. 62*: 295-308.

O'Malley, B.W. and Means, A.R. (1974). *Science 183*: 610-620.

O'Malley, B.W., Sherman, M.R., and Taft, D.O. (1970). *Proc. Natl. Acad. Sci. USA 67*: 501-508.

Puca, G.A., Sica, V., and Nola, E. (1974). *Proc. Natl. Acad. Sci. USA 71*: 979-983.

Radley, J.M. (1968). *Exp. Cell Res. 48*: 679-681.

Robbins, S.L. 1962). Pathology. W.B. Saunders, Philadelphia, p. 21.

Sandritter, W. and Adler, C.P. (1971). *Experientia 27*: 1435-1437.

Sandritter, W. and Scomazzoni, G. (1964). *Nature 202*: 100-101.

Schneyer, C.A., Finley, W.H., and Finley, S.C. (1967). *Proc. Soc. Exp. Biol. Med. 125*: 722-728.

Spelsberg, T.C., Steggles, A.W., and O'Malley, B.W. (1971). *J. Biol. Chem. 246*: 4188-4197.

Steggles, A.W., Spelsberg, T.C., Glasser, S.R., and O'Malley, B.W. (1971). *Proc. Natl. Acad. Sci. USA 68*: 1479-1482.

Studzinski, G.P. and Gierthy, J.F. (1973). *J. Cell. Physiol. 81*: 71-84.

Swartz, F., Sams, B.F., and Barton, A.G. (1960). *Exp. Cell Res. 20*: 438-446.

Szirmai, J.A. (1962). In *Protein Metabolism F. Gross (Ed.). Springer Verlag,*

Szirmai, J.A. (1962). In *Protein Metabolism*, F. Gross (Ed.). Springer Verlag, Heidelberg, p. 45.

Tata, J.R. (1968). *Nature 219*: 331-337.

Tata, J.R. (1970). *Biochem J. 116*: 617-630.

Toniolo, D., Meiss, H.K., and Basilico, C. (1973). *Proc. Natl. Acad. Sci. USA 70*: 1273-1277.

Winick, M. and Noble, A. (1965). *Dev. Biol. 12*: 451-466.

THIRTEEN

THE CANCER CELL

Before we discuss the molecular basis of neoplastic transformation, let us summarize what has been said thus far about the normal cell of the adult animal. We have seen that cells in the adult body can be divided into three large categories: (a) differentiated cells, that is, cells destined to die without dividing again; (b) cells that ordinarily do not divide and do not synthesize DNA but can be stimulated to do so by an appropriate stimulus; and (c) continuously dividing cells that move around the cell cycle from one mitosis to the next one. We have seen that in the latter category of cells the biochemical events occurring between one mitosis and the next proceed in an orderly fashion and are programmed in roughly the same way as they are in the cell cycle of bacterial cells. Although gene products are certainly involved in the regulation of the flow of cells through the cell cycle, the evidence is not as abundant as in G_0 cells stimulated to proliferate. After the earthquake of mitosis, the cells pull themselves together, the preexisting messenger RNA again shifts to polysomes from a masked form, and a number of steps involving protein and RNA synthesis occur, which eventually lead to the onset of DNA synthesis. After completion of DNA synthesis, another series of steps, again involving the synthesis of specific proteins and specific RNA molecules, lead to mitosis.

In the second category of cells, which we now identify as G_0 cells, the sequence of events changes after a certain number of mitoses and the cells become quiescent. We have little or no information on what causes a cell to leave the cycle and become a G_0 cell, but we do have a considerable amount of information on the sequence of biochemical events that occur when G_0 cells are stimulated to proliferate by an appropriate stimulus. The triggering event is activation of the genome as measured by functional and structural changes in chromatin. This activation is preceded by a number of events, which are genome independent and in which certain nonhistone chromosomal proteins play an important role. After the increase in transcriptional activity of chromatin and in membrane transport function, the biochemical events in stimulated G_0 cells are very similar to those described in the G_1 period of continuously dividing cells.

TUMOR GROWTH AT THE CELLULAR LEVEL

We have also seen that any tissue grows, at a cellular level, on the basis of variations in the following three parameters described in previous chapters: (a) the length of the cell cycle in the fraction of cells that continuously divide; (b) the growth fraction, that is, the fraction of cells that are in the cell cycle; and (c) the rate of cell loss. Under hormonal or other influences a tissue can grow and increase the total number of cells by either shortening the length of the cell cycle, recruiting cells from the G_0 fraction, or reducing the rate of cell loss. These three mechanisma are all very important, and in most cases they are all operative in determining the increase in cell number of a given cell population.

It does not take a profound observer to realize that cancer is a disturbance of growth, although apparently it does take an experienced observer to realize that not all disturbances of growth are cancer. This has caused a considerable amount of confusion in the past 20 years since the behavior of certain cells in culture has often been interpreted as neoplastic transformation by investigators who chose to overlook the characteristics of cancer growth. Thus, the fact that some cells can reach a higher saturation density when plated as a monolayer in cell cultures does not necessarily equate with neoplastic transformation and this is important to keep in mind if we really wish to understand the molecular basis of the neoplastic transformation. In fact, if we remember, as mentioned above, that cancer is a disturbance of growth but that not all such disturbances are cancer, we can probably have a better understanding of the situation and explain some of the disappointments that have occurred when some of the results obtained in cell cultures have been transferred to the living animal.

In the first place at a cellular level cancer is characterized by an increase in cell number. As previously mentioned, any tissue can increase the number of cells in the population by one of three ways: (a) shortening the cell cycle, (b) increasing the growth fraction by recruiting G_0 cells into the cell cycle, and (c) decreasing the rate of cell loss. The first report that cancer cells do not necessarily proliferate faster than do normal cells appeared in 1962 when Baserga and Kisieleski showed that there are certain normal cells in the adult animal whose cell cycle is shorter than that of even the fastest growing tumors. Thus, it became apparent from their data that the increase in cell number that accompanies the production of a tumor in an animal depended on factors other than simple shortening of the cell cycle. From the subsequent works of a number of investigators, which have been summarized in some recent reviews by Bresciani (1965), Steel et al. (1966), and Baserga and Wiebel (1969), it has become apparent that tumors grow by a combination of all three parameters mentioned above. ie., by decreasing the length of the cell cycle in respect to normal cells of the tissue of origin, by increasing the growth fraction (i.e., by recruiting a number of G_0 cells into the proliferating pool), and even by reducing the rate of cell loss. The most prominent mechanism is recruiting G_0 cells into the proliferating pool, and it has, in fact, become clear from a number of recent investigations in animals and man that growing tumors usually have a higher growth fraction than their normal counterpart tissue (Gavosto and Pileri 1971). This is important because it clearly indicates that cancer is not simply the neoplastic transformation of continuously dividing cells into cells that go from one mitosis to the next at a faster pace than their normal counterparts, but that, on the contrary, cancer is a problem of lack of control in the growth fraction, that is, of a lack of control in the number of cells that participate in the proliferation pool. The problem can be turned around and put it into these terms: in a normal tissue the number of cells in the population reaches a maximum, after which there is a balance (steady state) between the number of cells produced daily and the number that daily die. In certain conditions, especially hyperplasia, the balance is set somewhat higher, that is, there is an increase in the total number of cells but only up to another maximum. The balance is then restored and this keeps the total number of cells constant, although at a higher level than in the normal tissue of origin. In cancer no balance is ever reached, and the daily production of cells is always above the rate of cell loss. As mentioned above, this is essentially accomplished not by shortening the length of the cell cycle but by incresing the growth fraction, ie., the number of cells in the proliferating pool. What is failing in cancer is, therefore, the control mechanism that regulates the social behavior of cells in tissues and maintains the growth fraction characteristic of the normal tissue of origin. As an illustration, we give, in Table 13.1, some data carefully collected by Bresciani et al. (1974) and by Iversen et al. (1974) on human tumors. Several interesting things can be gleaned from the data, namely: (a) in most cases the S phase is rather long, 18 hours or more, the only exception being the Burkitt lymphoma; (b) the actual doubling time (observed time necessary for a tumor to double its size) is always much longer than its potential doubling time (which is the length of the cell cycle if *all* cells divided and *no* cells died); (c) the growth fraction is always lower than 100% and is lowest in the slowest growing tumors; and (d) the number of new cells produced per unit time always exceeds the number of cells lost per unit time. The last two columns in Table 13.1 indeed summarize, in the most succinct way, why tumors grow.

If growth in cancer is deranged, one may legitimately ask what is the molecular basis of this altered control.

Table 13.1   Growth of Human Tumors

Tumor	Cell cycle (T_c; hr)	S phase (T_s; hr)	Doubling time (days)	Growth fraction (%)	Cell birth rate[a]	Cell loss rate[b]
Squamous Cell Carcinomas of Head[c]						
Patient No. 1	62	18	13	62	100	78
Patient No. 2	62	18	25	39	61	50
Patient No. 3	72	28	107	31	43	40
Patient No. 4	52	21	18	45	86	70
Patient No. 5	72	19	34	45	63	55
Patient No. 6	61	26	12	84	138	114
Patient No. 7	88	34	68	41	47	43
Burkitt Lymphoma[d]	25.6	6.5	2¾	85	85	69

[a]Number of cells produced per hour and 10^4 cells.
[b]Number of cells disappearing from tissue per hour and 10^4 cells.
[c]From Bresciani et al. (1974).
[d]From Iversen et al. (1974).

PROGRESSION OF TUMORS

We are not concerned here with the causes of cancer in terms of exogenous causes, nor with neoplastic growth as such, the immunological reaction it causes, the clinical symptoms it produces, and eventually its ability to spread all over the body as metastatic growths. The only thing that we are concerned with here are changes at the molecular level that cause the initially transformed cancer cell to escape the regulatory mechanisms for cell proliferation. Recent evidence, summarized by Fialkow (1972), indicates that most cancers in man are of clonal origin, that is, they originate from a single transformed cell. It would be a mistake to think that identification of the molecular basis responsible for initial neoplastic transformation can explain the whole natural history of cancer. On the contrary, a considerable amount of evidence (summarized by Good 1972) also indicates that transformed cancer cells in man as well as in the adult animal undergo a continuous immunological surveillance, which causes most of the initially transformed neoplastic cells to die. Only in a few instances do the transformed cancer cells survive and establish a neoplastic growth which eventually becomes clinically detectable. Thus, it is quite possible that the initial transformation results, in a great majority of cases, in a cell promptly eliminated by the defense mechanisms of the body, especially by immunological defenses. It is also possible that in a number of cases, cancer cells may grow at a slower pace till they reach a certain stage where a successive progression of changes, perhaps abetted by a DNA polymerase lacking the appropriate fidelity (Springgate and Loeb 1973), leads to markedly anaplastic cells with a variety of growth disturbances. Thus, by the time a cancer becomes widespread in the human body, it is likely that different clones of cells may have developed. In some clones the cell cycle may have been shortened drastically in respect to the normal counterpart and the lack of growth control may extend way beyond the initial transformation, simply involving a derangement of growth control at the level of the growth fraction. For instance, the immunological status of the host affected growth rate and rate of cell loss but not the length of the cell cycle

in three transplantable rat tumors (Janik and Steel 1972). The
natural history of some of these tumors has been described in a very
accurate way in a specific tumor of man, melanoma of the skin, and
the reader could benefit considerably by reading the work of Clark
and collaborators (1971) on this subject. What we would like to
discuss here is the molecular change that leads to the initial lack of
growth control.

THE CASE OF XERODERMA PIGMENTOSUM

Since we know now that control of cellular proliferation resides at the gene level and that possibly in a series of genes
specifically controlling the initiation of DNA synthesis and cell
division, one would have to postulate that the initial molecular
lesion leading to the initial neoplastic transformation must reside
in genes that control cellular proliferation. Two kinds of mechanisms
can be considered here, and they will be examined in detail separately. The first is a possible lesion at the nucleotide level caused by
an exogenous agent. As an illustration of such a mechanism, consider the disease *Xeroderma pigmentosum.*

Xeroderma pigmentosum is a rare and very serious hered-
itary disease of the skin, possibly caused by an autosomal recessive
gene and characterized by hypersensitivity of the epidermis to sunlight or ultraviolet light. It usually develops in childhood, sometimes in the first year of life. The skin develops lesions similar to
those seen in chronic radiation dermatitis. Pigmented macules
that look like ordinary freckles appear, and in the later stages the
skin is dry and atrophic, with mottled pigmentation. Histopath-
ologically there appears a combination of hyperkeratosis, marked
atrophy of the rete malpighii, dilatation of vessels, and a greatly increased accumulation of melanin. The eyes are affected and photo-
phobia and lacrimation may be intense. In addition there is a pronounced tendency to develop basal cells and epidermoid carcinomas
of the skin, which appear in large numbers over the course of

Table 13.2   **Thymidine Index of Human Skin Fibroblasts
after Various Doses of Ultraviolet Light**

	Control (%)	100 erg/mm^2 (%)	500 erg/mm^2 (%)	1,000 erg/mm^2 (%)
Normal	41.2	100	100	100
Ataxia telang.	23.1	100	100	100
Xeroderma pig.	24.2	25.3	24.6	27.4
do.	19.0	23.2	21.0	15.0
do.	22.2	28.9	29.2	26.0

[a]From Cleaver, J.E. (1968).

years. Various other forms of benign and malignant tumors of ecto-dermal and mesodermal origin also occur with a much increased frequency in affected individuals. All of these abnormalities appear to be the consequence of over-exposure to sunlight. Cleaver, in 1968, showed that the extreme sensitivity of individuals with *Xeroderma pigmentosum* to ultraviolet light could be explained by a defect in their mechanism for DNA repair. Cleaver (1968) cultured human skin fibroblasts from normal individuals and from individuals with *Xeroderma pigmentosum* and exposed them to an ultraviolet light predominantly of a 2537 Å wavelength. The cells treated with ultraviolet light were then exposed to tritiated thymidine and the number of labeded cells was counted. The results are shown in Table 13.2. About 40% of normal skin fibroblasts in culture are in DNA synthesis at any given time. After exposure to ultraviolet light, fibroblasts not in the S phase undergo unscheduled DNA synthesis so that 100% of them become labeled with tritiated thymidine. Skin fibroblasts cultured from a patient with a skin disorder called *ataxia telangiectasia* behave very much like the skin fibroblasts from normal individuals. However, when skin fibroblasts from patients with *Xeroderma pigmentosum* are cultured, notice that the number of cells labeled with tritiated thymidine is essentially the same in controls and in

cells exposed to ultraviolet light, meaning that in these cells DNA
repair does not occur or occurs to such a small extent that it is not
detectable by ordinary autoradiographic methods. This was a very
exciting result since it indicated that the extreme sensitivity of the
skin of these patients to ultraviolet light could be correlated to a
specific molecular mechanism, that is, their inability to repair DNA,
and possibly that this inability could be correlated to the very high
incidence of squamous cell carcinoma in the skin of these patients.
Later Cleaver (1969) extended these studies in an attempt to identify
the enzymatic defect in patients with Xeroderma pigmentosum. He
took advantage of the difference in the type of damage in DNA caused
by ultraviolet light or x-rays. He showed that fibroblasts from patients
with homozygous Xeroderma pigmentosum could perform repair replication after chain breakage caused by x-ray, but not after ultraviolet
damage. The final step in this interesting series of investigations was
reported by Epstein and coworkers (1970) who studied the DNA repair mechanism directly in skin cells. They found that when normal
human skin is exposed in vivo to ultraviolet irradiation at wavelengths
shorter than 320 nm unscheduled DNA synthesis was stimulated in
all cell layers of the epidermis and in the upper dermal fibrocytes.
The skin of patients with Xeroderma pigmentosum did not show
this response. These studies then indicate that structural damage to
DNA can be repaired by repair mechanisms and in certain patho-
logical conditions the main defect may possibly be the inability to
repair the damage. It is also conceivable that the lesion induced by
ultraviolet rays resides in the nucleotide sequence that controls
cellular proliferation. Many other mutations may be caused by
ultraviolet light in cells of patients with Xeroderma pigmentosum,
mutations that are due to the inability of the cells of the patients
with such a disease to repair the lesion. Most of the mutations will
have nothing to do with cancer, since some will simply cause death
of cells because they involve certain genes whose products are necessary to the life processes of the cell. In many other cases, the mutation may reside in other genes that are not expressed in that particular
cell. As already mentioned, most of the genes in mammalian cells
are repressed. Therefore, a mutation in a gene that is not expressed

in a particular cell will not be detected. For instance, in an epidermal cell a mutation induced in the genes that control the synthesis of myoglobin will be undetectable. Thus, of the many mutations, some totally insignificant and others lethal, only a few will result in a cancerous transformation because they will directly involve the nucleotide sequence that controls the initiation of cell proliferation. It should be mentioned here that there is considerable evidence that many physical and chemical carcinogens are also mutagenic. In my opinion, the most clever experiment in support of chemical mutation in cancer comes from Tomatis and Goodall (1969) who injected pregnant mice with the carcinogen 7, 12-dimethylbenz (A) anthacene and found an increased incidence of tumors in the F_2 descendants (see also the review by Tomatis (1973) on tumor incidence in offspring of experimental animals exposed to carcinogens).

VIRAL TRANSFORMATION

The second possibility is the insertion of a viral genome in the genome of the mammalian cell. The evidence in favor of a viral etiology for many animal tumors and for some human tumors is increasing very rapidly. A review of the various viruses that can cause neoplastic transformation in mammalian cells can be found in Green (1970). The work of Spiegelman and collaborators (Axel et al. 1972, Kufe et al. 1972, 1973), has clearly indicated that gene sequences analogous to certain sequences in oncogenic animal viruses can be found in mammalian cells and, more especially, in tumor cells from human origin. The evidence also indicates that in the great majority of cases, at least, the viral genome is integrated in the genome of mammalian cells that have been transformed. However, some disturbing reports have appeared indicating that multiple copies of the viral genome can be found in transformed cells (Varmus et al. 1972). Even worse, some phenotypically normal BALB/3T3 cells, abortively transformed with SV-40 were found to contain five viral genome equivalents per diploid cell (Smith et al. 1972). In fact, mouse mammary tumor virus-specific nucleotide sequences are present in the DNA of both high and low tumor incidence mouse strains. Large amounts of virus-specific RNA are present in both virus-producing tumors and in lactating mammary glands (Varmus et al. 1973). The explanation for this phenomenon, which at first seems to invalidate the theory of the viral etiology of certain tumors, may be found in the experiment of Lindahl et al. (1971), who showed that the insertion of a phage genome in the bacterial genome must take place at a specific position in the circular DNA molecule in order to exert its effect. Lindahl et al. (1971), used a temperature-sensitive mutant of *E. coli* K 12 that is incapable of initiating DNA synthesis at the nonpermissive temperature, although it can grow and carry out DNA synthesis regularly at the permissive temperature. When this temperature-sensitive mutant *E. coli* is infected with prophage P2, certain phage-infected cells capable of growing at the nonpermissive temperature can be rescued. Lindahl et al. (1971), however, found that only a few of the temperature-sensitive mutants of *E. coli* were capable of growing at the nonpermissive temperature when infected with P2 prophage, and by genetic analysis they found that the strains in which the ability to grow at the nonpermissive temperature was restored contained P2 genome at a specific place in the DNA-circular molecule, that is, near the methionine gene. These experiments showed that while the P2 prophage genome may restore the ability of a bacterial cell to initiate DNA synthesis, it does so only when it is inserted at a specific place in the genome. The same may happen in viral transformation of mammalian cells, that is, cells are transformed only when the viral genome is integrated at a specific place in the genome of mammalian cells. This explains why viral genomes can be found in untransformed cells or why multiple copies of viral genomes can be found in untransformed cells or why multiple copies of viral genomes can be found in transformed cells.

In both cases of Xeroderma pigmentosum and of viral oncogenesis, it seems, therefore, that neoplastic transformation may be caused by an alteration in the nucleotide sequence occurring at a certain specific site in the genome of mammalian cells. It is also naturally tempting to speculate that the specific site is the same site that regulates cell proliferation in normal cells and that is activated when quiescent cells are stimulated to proliferate by an appropriate stimulus. This is indeed the theory that has been put forward by Comings (1973) in his very interesting general theory of carcinogenesis. Comings (1973) postulates the existence of *Tr* genes, which are permanently expressed in transformed cells but are only temporarily expressed in normal cells and that only when cells are proliferating. These genes are usually repressed by the product of an *i* gene (suppressing locus). Derangement in the control of cell proliferation could be caused by any mutation in *Tr* or *i* genes. Comings (1973) even proposes that the idea that oncogenic viruses are simply excised *Tr* genes.

Genetic differences between normal and transformed cells should lead to differences in chromatin and nonhistone chromosomal proteins. Indeed, several reports have appeared indicating differences in chromatin and nonhistone chromosomal proteins between normal cells and their transformed counterparts. These are listed in Table 13.3. It would be tempting to speculate that these differences derive from differences in chromosome C7, which seems to be necessary for imparting unlimited growth potential to hybrids from SV-40 transformed cells and cells with limited growth potential (Croce and Koprowski 1974). Whether or not an alteration of chromosome C7 is the basis of loss of growth control in cancer cells, the data in Table 13.3 show that there are impressive differences between normal and neoplastic cells in the chromosomal proteins that presumably regulate gene expression. Other differences at the molecular level have been reported between normal and transformed cells, and among these can be cited sensitivity to aminonucleoside (Cholon and Studzinski 1974b), cytochalasin B (Wright and Hayflick 1972, Kelly and Sambrook 1973), or bromodeoxyuridine (Grady and North 1974), ability to bind acridine orange after stimulation (Smets 1973), and differences in membrane structure and function as already discussed in chapter 9. However, changes in chromosomal proteins may be more pronounced than in extranuclear proteins, since regulation of one gene usually is under the influence of more than one protein.

Table 13.3   **Reported Differences in Chromatin and Non-histone Chromosomal Proteins between Normal and Transformed Cells**

Cell types	Differences in	References
WI-38 and 2RA (SV-40)	Chromatin	Lin et al. (1974)
WI-38 and 2RA	NHCP	Cholon and Studzinski (1974a)
Rat liver and Novikoff hepatoma	NHCP	Yeoman et al. (1973)
Rat liver and hepatoma 5123C	NHCP	Arnold et al. (1973)
Normal and neopl. mammary gland	NHCP	Kadohama and Turkington
gland	NHCP	(1973)
Lymphocytes and leukemic cells	NHCP	Weisenthal and Ruddon (1973)
Liver and hepatomas	NHCP	Wakabayashi and Hnilica (1973)
WI-38 and 2RA	NHCP	Zardi et al. (1973)
WI-38 and 2RA	NHCP	Krause and Stein (1974)
Brain cells and		Biessmann and Rajewsky
neuroectodermal tumors	NHCP	(1975)

In conclusion, after the initial transformation the neo-plastic cell still has a long way to go before it becomes an established, clinically detectable neoplasm, and it is quite possible that al-though neoplastic transformations may occur continuously in the body every day, most of the initially transformed cancer cells are continuously eliminated. It would, therefore, appear that establish-ment of a clinically detectable cancer is due to a complex number of factors, which include external causes, a change in a specific site of the genome, immunological surveillance, and tumor pro-gression. However, the natural history of cancer can be better studied in other texts, and we can, therefore, conclude our dis-cussion with the hope that the reader may have now gained a better understanding of factors that control normal and abnormal cellular proliferation in mammalian cells.

References

Arnold, E.A., Buksas, M.M., and Young, K.E. (1973). *Cancer Res. 33*: 1169-1176.

Axel, R., Schlom, J., and Spiegelman, S. (1972). *Proc. Natl. Acad. Sci. USA 69*: 535-538.

Baserga, R. and Kisieleski, W.E. (1962). *J Natl. Cancer Inst. 28*: 331-339.

Baserga, R. and Wiebel, F. (1969). *Int. Rev. Exp. Pathol. 7*: 1-30.

Biessmann, H. and Rajewsky, M.F. (1975). *J. Neurochem. 24*: 387-393.

Bresciani, F. (1965). *Cellular Radiation Biology*. M.D. Anderson Hospital Symposium, Williams and Wilkins, Baltimore, pp. 547-557.

Bresciani, F., Paoluzi, R., Benassi, M., Nervi, C., Casale, C., and Ziparo, E. (1974). *Cancer Res. 34*: 2405-2415.

Cholon, J.J. and Studzinski, G.P. (1974a). *Cancer Res. 34*: 588-593.

Cholon, J.I. and Studzinski, G.P. (1974b). *Science 184*: 160-161.

Clark, W.H. Jr. and Mihm, M.C. (1971). In *Dermatology in General Medicine,* T.B. Fitzpatrick et al. (eds.). McGraw-Hill, New york, pp. 491-511.

Cleaver, J.E. (1968). *Nature 218*: 652-656.

Cleaver, J.E. (1969). *Proc. Natl. Acad. Sci. 63*: 428-435.

Comings, D.E. (1973). *Proc. Natl. Acad. Sci. USA 70*: 3324-3328.

Croce, C.M. and Koprowski, H. (1974). *Science 184*: 1288-1289.

Epstein, J.H., Fukuyama, K., Reed, W.B., and Epstein, W.L. (1970). *Science 168*: 1477-1478.

Fialkow, P.K. (1972). *Adv. Cancer Res. 15*: 191-226.

Gavosto, F. and Pileri, A. (1971). In *The Cell Cycle and Cancer*, R. Baserga (Ed.). Marcel Dekker, New York, pp. 99-138.

Good, R.A. (1972). *Proc. Natl. Acad. Sci. USA 69*: 1026-1032.

Grady, L.J. and North, A.B. (1974). *Exp. Cell Res. 87*: 120-126.

Green, M. (1970). *Ann. Rev. Biochem. 39*: 701-756.

Iversen, O.H., Iversen, U., Ziegler, J.L., and Bluming, A.Z. (1974). *Eur. J. Cancer 10*: 155-163.

Janik, R. and Steel, G.G. (1972). *Br. J. Cancer 26*: 108-114.

Kodohama, N. and Turkington, R.W. (1973). *Cancer Res. 33*: 1194-1201.

Kelly, F. and Sambrook, J. (1973). *Nature New Biol. 242*: 217-219.

Krause, M.D. and Stein, G.S. (1974). *Biochem. Biophys. Res. Comm. 59*: 796-803.

Kufe, D., Hehlman, R., and Spiegelman, S. (1972). *Science 175*: 182-185.
Kufe, D., Hehlman, R., and Spiegelman, S. (1973). *Proc. Natl. Acad. Sci. USA 70*: 5-9.
Lin, J.C., Nicolini, C., and Baserga, R. (1974). *Biochemistry 13*: 4127-4133.
Lindahl, G., Hirota, Y., and Jacob, F. (1971). *Proc. Natl. Acad. Sci. USA 68*: 2407-2411.
Smets, L.A. (1973). *Exp. Cell Res. 79*: 239-243.
Smith, H.S., Gelb, L.D., and Martin, M.A. (1972). *Proc. Natl. Acad. Sci. USA 69*: 152-156.
Springgate, C.F. and Loeb, L.A. (1973). *Proc. Natl. Acad. Sci. USA 70*: 245-249.
Steel, G.G., Adams, K., and Barrett, J.C. (1966). *Br. J. Cancer 20*: 784-800.
Tomatis, L. and Goodall, C.M. (1969). *Int. J. Cancer 4*: 219-225.
Tomatis, L. (1973). In *Modern Trends in Oncology*, R. W. Raven (Ed.). Butterworth, London, pp. 99-126.
Varmus, H.E., Weiss, R.A., Freis, R.R., Levinson, W., and Bishop, J.M. (1972). *Proc. Natl. Acad. Sci. USA 69*: 20-24.
Varmus, H.E., Quintrell, H., Medeiros, E., Bishop, G.M., Nowinski, R.C., and Sarkar, N.H. (1973). *J. Mol. Biol. 79*: 663-679.
Wakabayshi, K. and Hnilica, L.S. (1973). *Nature New Biol. 242*: 153-155.
Weisenthal, L.M. and Ruddon, R.W. (1973). *Cancer Res. 33*: 2923-2935.
Wright, W.E. and Hayflick, L. (1972). *Exp. Cell Res. 74*: 187-194.
Yeoman, L.C., Taylor, C.W., Jordan, J.J., and Busch, H. (1973). *Biochem. Biophys. Res. Comm. 53*: 1067-1076.
Zardi, L., Lin, J. C., and Baserga, R. (1973). *Nature New Biol. 244*: 211-213.

AUTHOR INDEX

Italic numbers give the page on which the complete reference is listed.

A

Abelson, H. T., 101, *102*, 194, *198*
Abercrombie, M., 146-147, *156*
Abrams, R., 22, *28*, 44, 50, *52*, 57, 63, *75*, 81, *104*, 181, *187*
Abrass, I. R., 83, *105*
Adams, K., 12, *16*, 202, *214*
Adams, R. L. P., 22, *28*, 181, *187*
Adelberg, E. A., 36, *42*
Adelman, R. C., 180, *187*
Adler, C. P., 191, *198, 199*
Ahern, T., 141, *145*
Ahmed, K., 68, *75*, 133, *145*
Aimar, C., 6, *15*
Alberts, B. M., 23, *28*
Albright, M. L., 167, *173*
Allfrex, V. G., 33, *42*, 82, 88, *105*, 101, *102*, 108-111, 114, 117, 119-120, *125-130*, 137, *144-145*, 185, *187*, 194, *198*
Aloni, Y., 100, *102*, 138, *144*

Alvarez, M. R., 94-95, *102,* 196, *198*
Ambrose, E. J., 146-147, *156*
Amodio, F. J., 23, *28*
Amos, H., 141, *145*
Andrews, H., 148, *158*
Anderson, E. C., 32-33, 35, *42*
Anderson, K. M., 89, *103,* 120, *126*
Anderson, S. L., 114, *129*
Anderson, W. B., 67, *76*
Angerer, L. M., 95, *102*
Antoniades, H. N., 166, *173*
Appels, R., 110, *126*, 137, *144*, 185, *187*
Appleton, D., 35, *43*
Argyris, T. S., 34, *41*
Ariake, S., 21, *30*
Armstrong, N. B., 58, *77*
Armstrong, N. D., 166, 168, *174*
Armstrong, R. L., 54, *73*
Arnason, B. G. W., 135, *144*
Arnold, E. A., 114, *126*, 212, *213*
Ashburner, M., 70, *73*

Atkins, M., 141, *145*
Atlas, M., 27, *28*, 35, *41*, 50, *51*
Auer, G., 95, *106*, 137, *144*
Augenlicht, L., 86, *102*, 180, 184, *187*
Augenlicht, L. H., 114, 124, *126*
Avery, O. T., 2, *15*
Axel, R., 88, *102*, 209, *213*
Aye, M. T., 166, *174*

B

Baker, R. M., 79, *106*
Balhorn, R., 47, *51*
Bank, A., 63, *76*, 82, *104*
Bannai, S., 88, *102*
Barbiroli, B., 154, *156*, 183, *187*
Barka, T., 7, *15*, 55, 58-59, 61, *73*
Barker, K. L., 85, 88-89, *102*, 142-143, *145*
Barnoux, C., 19, *29*
Barrett, J. C., 12, *16*, 202, *214*
Barrett, T., 114-115, *126*
Barton, A. G., 193, *199*
Baseman, J. P., 143, *144*
Baserga, R., 3,11,13,*15*, 21-22-26, *28*, *30*, 34-35, 37-39, *41-42*, 44-47, 49-50, *51-52*, 53, 55-56, 58-69, 72, *73-77*, 82-83, 86, 89-97, 101, *102-105*, 108-109, 111-114, 116-118, 120-124, *126*, *129-130*, 131-132, 135, 137-138, 143, *144-155*, 154, *157-158*, 167, *172*, 177-178, 180-185, *187-188*, 192, 197, *198-199*, 202, 212, *213-214*
Basilico, C., 48, *51*, 67, *73*, 79-80, *103*, *106*,197, *199*
Bates, C. J., 164, *172*
Baulie, E., 155, *158*
Baxter, J. D., 139-140, *145*

Becker, F. F., 177, *187*
Becker, H., 121, *126*, 141, *144*, 181, 187, 197, *198*
Becker, Y., 56, *73*, 185, *188*
Bekhor, I., 114, *126*
Bell, B. M., 27, *29*, 35, *42*
Benassi, M., 203-204, *213*
Ben-Bassat, H., 149, *158*
Berger, N. A., 56, *73*
Bergeron, J. J. M., 152, *158*
Bernhard, W., 148, *158*
Bertram, J. S., 47-48, *51*
Bessler, W., 56, *76*
Betel, I., 154-155, *159*
Biessmann, H., 212, *213*
Billing, R. J., 154, *156*, 183, *187*
Birnstiel, M. L., 22, *29*
Bishop, G. M., 210, *214*
Bishop, J. M., 209, *214*
Bissell, M. J., 143, *144*
Blat, C., 120, *127*, 134, *144*
Blenkinsopp, W. K., 27, *28*
Blobel, G., 141, *145*
Blumfeld, O. O., 56, *77*
Bluming,A. Z., 203-204, *213*
Boffa, L. C., 114, *130*
Boivin, A., 5, *15*
Bolle, A., 70, *76*
Bolund, L.,86-87, 93-95, *102-103*, *105*, 123-124, *126*, 136-137, *144-145*, 185, *187*
Bombik, B. M., 66, *73*, 92, 94, 100, *102-103*
Bond, V. P., 21, 27, *28-29*, 35, *41*, 50, *51*
Bonner, J., 71, *75*, 84-86, 88, 94, *103-104*, 109, 112, 114, 116, 121, *126-127*,*129*
Boone, C. W., 185, *188*
Boone, R. F., 83, *105*
Bordwell, J., 47, *51*
Borun, T., 18, *30*, 60, *77*

Borun, T. W., 25-26, *28*, *30*, 33, *42*, 47, *51-52*, 113, *126*
Bosmann, H. B., 148, *157*
Bostok, C. J., 23, *28*
Bourne, R. A., 58, *73*
Boutwell, R. K., 58, *75*
Bradbury, E. M., 33, *41*
Brade, W. P., 68, *73*, 89, *103*, 133, *144*
Brady, R. O., 149, *157*
Brailovsky, C., 148, 150, *157-158*
Branton, P. E., 149, *159*
Braun, R., 28, *29*
Bray, G., 22, *28*
Breckenridge, B. M., 66, *73*
Brent, T. P., 22, *28*, 47, *51*
Bresciani, F., 27, *28*, 50, *51*, 58, *73*, 202-204, *213*
Briggs, R., 6, *15*
Brittinger, G., 89, *104*
Broome, J. D., 177, *187*
Brown, D. F., 32, *41*
Brown, R. F., 168, *174*
Bruchovsky, N., 58, *75*
Brumbaugh, P. F., 153, *157*
Brutlag, D., 21, *31*
Bryant, J. A., 58, *73*
Bucher, N. L. R., 55, 58, 61, *73*, 167, *172*, 180, *187*
Buchowicz, J., 70, *74*
Buck, A. T., 53, 58, 77, 82, *105*
Buck, C. A., 36, *41*, 151, *157*
Buck, M. D., 117, *126*
Buckingham, M. E., 71, *73*
Buell, D., 18, *28*, 47, *51*
Buksas, M. M. 212, *213*
Bullough, W. S., 34, *41*, 169, *172*
Burdette, K. E., 25, *28*
Burdzy, K., 58, *76*
Burger, M. M., 36, *41*, 56, 66, 71, *73*, *76*, 146-149, 151-152, *157*, *159*, 165, *172*

Burk, R. R., 56, 72, *73*
Burstin, S. J., 48, *51*, 67, *73*, 80, *103*
Busch, H., 108, 113, *126*, 212, *214*
Bustin, M., 110, *126*
Butcher, F. R., 34, *41*, 67, *74*
Butler, J. A. V., 47, *51*, 108, *128*
Butler, P. J. G., 122, *126*
Butterworth, P. H. W., 87, *103*
Buttin, G., 80, *105*
Byrt, P., 62, *73*, 143, *144*

C

Cairns, J., 19, *28*
Campbell, J. L., 20, *30*
Campbell, R. D., 40, *41*
Campbell, W. P., 99, *104*
Caput, D., 71, *73*
Carbonell, A. W., 48, *52*
Carchman, R. A., 67, *76*
Carey, N. H., 89, 100, *103*
Carlsson, S., 136, 137, *144*, *145*
Carol, B., 58, *74*
Carroll, A., 116, *128*
Carter, D. B., 124, *126*
Casale, C., 203-204, *213*
Cave, MacD., 35, *41*
Ceder, H., 88, *102*
Chalkley, R. G., 18, 47, *51*, 86, *103*, 110, *128*
Chambon, P., 101, *103*
Chandrabose, K. A., 152, *157*
Chapman, R. E., 50, *51*
Chase, M., 2, *15*
Chaudhuri, S., 63, *73*, 121-122, *130*
Chelmicka-Szorc, E., 135, *144*
Cheng, R. F., 164-166, 170, *173*
Chesterton, C. J., 87, *103*
Chiu, H., 197, *198*
Chiu, J., 90, *103*, 119, *126*
Chiu, J. A., 68, *73*, 89, *103*, 133, *144*

Choe, B. K., 113, *126*, 137, *144*
Choe, C., 124, *126*
Choie, D. D., 58, *73*, 178, *187*
Cholon, J. J., 121, *126*, 211, 212, *213*
Chu, L., 117, *130*
Chung, L. W. K., 120, *126*
Church, R. B., 70-71, *74*, 98-99, 101, *103*
Chytil, F., 90, 94, 101, *104-105*, 116, 120-122, *126-127*, *129*, 155, *157*, 196, *198*
Ciarrocchi, G., 22, *30*
Ciba Foundation Symposium, 86, *103*, 107, *126*
Clark, W. H., Jr., 206, *213*
Clarkson, B., 12, *15*, 20, 27, *28*, *30*, 35, *41*, 167, *172*
Cleaver, J. E., 27, *28*, 35, *41*, 50, *51*, 207-208, *213*
Clever, U., 70, *74*, 111, *126*
Cochet-Meihac, M., 101, *103*
Coffey, D. S., 120, *126*
Cognetti, G., 121, *126*
Cohen, A., 71, *73*
Cohen, S., 57, *74*, 124, *127*, 141, *144*, 165, *172*
Cohn, Z., 186, *187*
Cole, R. D., 85, *105*, 108-110, 113, 120, *130*
Colot, H. V., 140, *145*
Colyer, R. A., 25, *28*
Comings, D. E., 24, *28*, 113, *126*, 211, *213*
Conner, J. D., 165, *172*
Cooper, H. L., 7, *15*, 55-56, 63, *74*, 82, *103*
Cooper, N. R., 47, *52*
Corneille, L., 170, *174*
Costlow, M., 46, 49, *51*, 154, 157, 177, 181-183, *187*
Couch, R. M., 89, *103*, 120, *126*

Courtois, Y., 121, *127*
Courvalin, J. C., 101, *103*
Cowdry, E. V., 1, 5-7, *15*
Cox, R. F., 87, 89, 100, *103*
Craddock, C., 90, *103*, 119, *126*
Crampton, C. F., 108, *127*
Crathorn, A. R., 47, *51*
Creuzet, C., 116, *128*
Crippa, M., 71, *74*
Critchley, D. R., 152, *157*
Croce, C. M., 57, *74*, 211, *213*
Crocker, T. T., 113, *127*
Croizat, H., 50, *51*
Cronkite, E. P., 27, *29-30*
Cross, M. L., 26, *28*, 114, *127*
Crueuzet, C., 116, *128*
Cuatrecasas, P., 57, *75*
Culotti, J., 14, *15*, 79, *104*
Cumar, F. A., 149, *157*
Cunningham, D. D., 22, *28*, 61, *74*, 83, *103*, 152, 154-156, *157*

D

Dahmus, M., 84, 86, *103*, 109, *126*
Dalpra, L., 22, *30*
Daly, M. M., 108, *127*
Darnell, G. E., 100, *103*
Darzynkiewicz, A., 93, 95, 98, 103, *105*, 135, *144*
Dastugue, B., 121, *127*
David, C. N., 40, *41*
Davies, D. D., 110, *129*
DeAsua, L. J., 153-154, 156, *157*
De Cosse, J. J., 9, *15*, 196, *198*
Defendi, V., 24, 27, *28*, *30*, 35, *41*, 56-57, 77, 120, *129*, 148, *158*, 163, 165-167, *172-173*
Deich, R. A., 24, *29*
DeLange, R. J., 108, 110, *127*

De La Torre, C., 20, *29*
Dell'Orco, R. T., 181, *187*
DeLucia, P., 19, *28*
DeMorales, M. M., 120, *127*, 134, *144*
Derge, J. G., 23, *29*
Deschamps, Y., 170, *174*
DeSombre, E. R., 195-196, *198*
Dethlefsen, L., 139-140, *145*
Dice, J. F., 113, *127*
Diez, J. L., 20, *29*
Dill, B. C., 110, *128*
Dillman, W., 114, *130*
Dina, D., 71, *74*
Dingman, C. W., 85-87, *103*, 110, 113, 116, *127*
DiPasquale, A., 34, *42*
Dixon, G. H., 87, *104*, 111, 113, 116, *128*, *130*
Dobrzanska, M., 70, *74*
Doi, O., 63, *73*
Doida, Y., 45, 47, 50, *51*
Downes, A. M., 50, *51*
Dulak, N. C., 57, *74*, 165-166, *172*
Dulbecco, R., 56, *74*, 79, *103*, 148, 153-154, 156, *157*, 171, *172*
Dunham, E., 67-68, *74*
Durham, J. P., 34, *41*, 67, *74*

E

Eagle, H., 160-161, *172*, 185, *188*
Eberle, H., 23, *30*
Eckhart, W., 79, *103*, 148, *157*
Edelman, G. M., 180, *187*
Edelman, I., 117, *130*
Ege, T., 136, *145*
Eisenstein, R., 197, *198*
Elgin, S. C. R., 85, *103*, 114, 116, *127*, *130*
Elkington, J., 171, *172*

Ellem, K. A. O., 63, *74*, 164, *172*
Ellgaard, E. G., 111, *126*
Emmelot, P., 149, *156*
Emerson, C. P. Jr., 186, *187*
Enea, V., 117, *127*
Engelhardt, D. L., 185, *187*
Englander, D., 180, *187*
Epifanova, O. I., 7-8, *15*, 50, *51*, 55, *74*, 177, 187, 195, *198*
Epstein, J. H., 208, *213*
Epstein, R., 70, *76*
Epstein, W. L., 208, *213*
Estensen, R. D., 44-45, 47, *51*, 67-68, *74*
Everson, L, K., 18, *28*

F

Fabrikant, J. I., 13, *15*, 27, *29*, 35, *41*
Fache, J., 27, *30*
Fahey, J. L., 47, *51*
Fakan, S., 24, *29*
Falaschi, A., 22, *30*
Falconer, I. R., 58, *73*
Fambrough, D., 84, 86, *103*, 109, *126*
Fan, H., 38, *41*
Farber, J., 38-39, *41-42*, 50, *51*, 55, 72, *73-74*, 82-83, 89-90, *103*, 111, 124, *126*, *129*, 131-132, *144-145*, 177, *183*, *187*
Faulkner, R., 110, *125*
Feinendegen, L. E., 3, *15*, 21, *29*
Felsenfeld, G., 88, *102*
Ferris, F. L., 23, *28*
Fialkow, P. K., 205, *213*
Fibach, E., 149, *158*
Fievez, M., 26, *31*
Finley, S. C., 192, *199*
Finley, W. H., 192, *199*

Firtel, R. A., 71, *74*, 100, *103*
Fischer, B., 191, *198*
Fisher, D. B., 142, *144*, 152, *157*
Fisher, H. W., 170, *174*
Fishman, P. H., 149, *157*
Fitzgerald, P. G., 58, *74*
Fleishman, R. A., 20, *30*
Fliedner, T. M., 27, *29-30*
Forrest, G. L., 25, *29*, 33, 34, *41-42*
Foster, D. O., 150-151, *157*
Fouquet, H., 28, *29*
Fox, M., 18, *30*, 36, *41*, 49, 51, 151, *157*, 181, *187*
Frank, W., 164-166, *172*
Frayssinet, C., 193, *198*
Freis, R. R., 209, *214*
Frenkel, G. D., 20, *30*
Friedman, D. L., 20, *29*, 180, *187*
Friedman, R. M., 67, *75*
Friend, C., 56, *74*
Frindel, E., 18, 27, *29*, 50, *51*
Froehlich, J. E., 66, *74*
Fry, R. J. M., 4, 10, *15*, 27, *29*, 35, *41*
Fujimura, F., 84, 86, *103*
Fujioka, M., 63, *74*, 82, *103*
Fukuda, M., 193, *198*
Fukuyama, K., 208, *213*
Furth, J. J., 87, *104*

G

Gabelman, N., 56, *74*
Gahmberg, C. G., 149, 150, *157-158*
Gallien, C., 6, *15*
Garrard, W. T., 108, 112, 114, 121, *127*
Garrels, J. I., 114, *127*
Garren, L. D., 58, *76*, 83, *105*
Gavosto, F., 12-13, *15*, 202, *213*
Gaza, D. J., 69, *74*

Geelen, J. L. M. C., 122, *128*
Gefter, M. L., 19, *29*
Gelb, L. D., 210, *214*
Gelbard, A. S., 47, *51*
Gelfant, S., 9, *15*, 40, *41*, 196, *198*
Getz, S., 90, *103*, 119, *126*
Gierthy, J. F., 197, *199*
Gilbertson, J. R., 168, *174*
Gilden, R. V., 150, *158*
Gill, D. M., 143, *144*
Gillespie D., 140, *145*
Gilmour, R. S., 85, 88, *104*, 115-116, 121, *127*, *129*
Gimenez-Martin, G., 20, *29*
Glasser, S. R., 101, *103*, 120, 127, 155, *157*, 195-196, *198-199*
Gledhill, B. L., 93, 98, *105*
Glick, M.C., 36, *41*, 151-152, *157*, *159*
Glynn, R. D., 155, *157*
Godman, G. C., 131, *145*
Goldberg, A. R., 36, *41*
Goldberg, N. D., 67-68, *74-75*
Goldstein, A. L., 56, *77*
Goldstein, I. J., 56, *76*
Goldstein, L., 136, *145*
Goldstone, M. B. A., 47, *52*
Gonzalez, E. M. 197, *198*
Gonzalez-Fernandez, A., 20, *29*
Gonzalez-Mujica, F., 116, *127*
Good, R. A., 205, *213*
Goodall, C. M., 209, *214*
Gordon, S., 186, *187*
Gorski, J., 153, *159*
Gospodarowicz, D., 165, *172*
Goto, S., 137, *144*, 185, *187*
Gottesfeld, J. M., 94, *104*
Gould, H., 87, *104*, 114-115, *126*
Grady, L. J., 99, *104*, 211, *213*
Graham, C. F., 136, *144*
Graham, J. M., 152, *157*
Granner, D., 47, *51-52*

Graziano, S. L., 114, *127*
Green, H., 7, *16*, 56, 63, 68, *74*, 76-77, 82, 92, 101, *102*, *104*, *106*, 197, *198*
Grimes, W. J., 67, *75*, 149-150, *157*
Grisham, J. W., 22, *29*, 50, *51*, 58, 75, 141, *145*, 167, *173*
Gronow, M., 114, *127*
Gros, F., 71, *73*
Gross, P. R., 140, *145*
Groves, C. M., 86, *106*
Grumbach, M. M., 24, *30*
Grzelczak, S., 70, *74*
Guillet, R., 6, *15*
Gunther, G. R., 180, *187*
Gurdon, J. B., 6, *15*, 22, *29*
Gurley, L. R., 25, *29*, 47-48, *52*
Gutman, E. D., 23, *28*

H

Hadden, E. M., 67-68, *74-75*
Hadden, J. W., 67-68, *74-75*
Haddox, M. K., 67-68, *74-75*
Haemmerli, G., 135, *145*, 169, *174*
Haines, M. E., 89, 100, *103*
Hakomori, S., 148-150, *157-158*
Hall, K., 166, *172*
Hall, S. H., 117, 124, *129*
Halvorson, H. O., 54, *75*
Hamilton, M. J., 85, *105*
Hamilton, T., 120, *130*
Hamilton, T. H., 7, *15*, 55, 58, 63, 75, 82, 85, 89, *104-105*, 195, *198*
Hampar, B., 23, *29*
Hanawalt, P. C., 24, *30*
Hancock, R., 24-25, *29*, 113, *127*
Hand, R., 24, *29*
Hanna, I. R. A., 50, *51*
Hardin, J. M., 25, *29*

Harding, C. V., 180, *187*
Harel, L., 120, *127*, 134, *144*
Harik, S. I., 69, *75*
Harris, H., 57, *75*, 93-95, *103*, 136, 139, *144*, 189, *198*
Hartwell, L. H., 14, *15*, 39-40, *41*, 56, 70, *74-75*, 79, *104*
Hatanaka, M., 150, *158*
Hatie, C., 143, *144*
Haussler, M. R., 153, *157*
Hayahishi, O., 114, *128*
Hayflick, L., 37, *43*, 211, *214*
Hävry, P., 148, *158*
Heby, O., 69, *75*
Hecht, L. I., 60, *75*
Heffler, S., 82, *102*
Hehlman, R., 209, *214*
Heidelberger, C., 47-48, *51*
Heidema, J., 116, *128*
Heidrick, M. L., 67, *75*
Heilbrunn, L. V., 36, *41*
Helmsing, P. J., 116, *127*
Henderson, J. Y., 33, *43*
Hennings, H., 34, *41*, 47, *51*, 58, *75*, 169, *173*
Hercules, K., 100, *104*
Hereford, L. M., 70, *75*
Herman, L., 58, *74*
Hershey, A. D., 2, *15*
Hershko, A., 183, *187*
Heywood, P., 50, *52*
Higa, A., 54, *75*
Hilborn, D. A., 150, *159*
Hildebrand, C. E., 47-48, *52*
Hill, B., 58, *75*, 101, *104*, 142, *145*
Hirokawa, Y., 56, *77*
Hirota, Y., 19, 20, *29*, 210, *214*
Hirshhorn, R., 89, *104*
Hnilica, L. S., 68, *73*, 86, 89-90, *103*, *106*, 108-109, 113, 115-116, 119, *126-129*, 133, *144*, 212, *214*
Hodge, L. D., 50, *51, 52*

Hodgson, G., 33, *42*, 58, *75*
Hoffman, R., 164-166, *172*
Hogan, B. L. M., 141, *144*
Hogg, N. M., 150, *158*
Hole, B. V., 167, *173*
Holland, J. J., 37-38, *42*, 183, *188*
Hollenberg, M. D., 57, 69, *75*
Holley, R. W., 162-163, 164, 165,
    171, *172, 173*
Holmes, D. S., 71, *75*
Holoubek, V., 113, *127*
Hoober, J. K., 124, *127*
Hood, L. E., 114, *127, 130*
Hooper, J. A., 110, *128*
Hori, T., 24, *29*
Houck, J. C., 34, *41*, 47, *51*, 164-
    166, 169-170, *173*
Hovi, T., 57, *77*, 165, *174*
Howard, A., 2, *15*
Huang, P. C., 121, *128*
Huang, R., 109, *126*
Huang, R. C., 84, 86, *103*, 114, 121,
    127-128
Huberman, J. A., 24, *29*, 39, *41*, 84,
    86, *103, 128*
Huebner, R. J., 150, *158*
Hughes, W. L., 21, *29*
Hugosson, R., 13, *16*, 57, *76*
Humphrey, R. M., 47, 49, *52*
Husakova, A., 168, *174*
Hynes, R. O., 149, *158*

I

Inbar, M., 148-149, *158*
Inglis, R. J., 33, *41*
Inoue, A., 137, *144*, 185, *187*
Ishida, H., 68, *75*, 133, *145*
Isselbacher, K., 155, *158*, 165-166,
    174
Iversen, O. H., 203-204, *213*

Iversen, U., 203-204, *213*

J

Jacob, F., 20, *29*, 78, *104*, 210, *214*
Jainchill, J. L., 162, 164, *173*
Janik, R., 206, *213*
Janne, J., 68, *76*
Jelinek, W. R., 100, *103*
Jenkins, M., 23, *28*
Jensen, E. V., 195-196, *198*
Jensen, R., 84, 86, *103*
Jentzsch, G., 25, *30*, 60, *76*
Jokusch, B. M., 32, *41*
Johns, E. W., 86-87, *102*, 108, 123-
    124, *126, 128*
Johnson, D. C., 37-38, *42*
Johnson, E. M., 33, *42*, 119, *128*,
    137, *144-145*, 185, *187*
Johnson, G. S., 67, *75-76*
Johnson, L. F., 101, *102*, 197, *198*
Johnson, R. T., 20, *30*, 34, *42*
Johnson, T. C., 183, *188*
Jokela, H. A., 108, 113, *128*
Jordan, J. J., 212, *214*
Jung, C., 47, *51*
Jungmann, R., 134, *145*

K

Kadohama, N., 212, *213*
Kaper, J. M., 122, *128*
Karn, J., 33, *42*, 119, *128*. 137, *144-
    145*, 185, *187*
Kay, J E., 68, *75*, 141, *145*, 152,
    158
Kelley, D. E., 49, *52*, 84, *105*
Kelley, F., 211, *213*
Kelly, F., 37, *42*, 211, *213*
Kember, N. F., 58, *75*

Keshgegian, A. A., 87, *104*
Kesse, M., 27, *29*
Kidwell, W. R., 25, *28*
Kiehn, D., 150, *157*
Kiernan, J. A., 162-163, 165, 171, *173*
Kijimoto, S., 149, *158*
Killander, D., 93-95, *105*
Kim, G., 114, *126*
Kim, J. H., 47, *51*
Kim, S., 110, *129*
King, J., *105*
King, R. J. B., 120, *129*
King, T. J., 6, *15*
Kish, V. M., 114, 116, *128-129*, 133, *145*
Kishimoto, S., 32, *42*
Kisieleski, W. E., 11, *15*, 202, *213*
Kleinsmith, L. J., 110, 114, 116, 119, 121, *128-130*, 133, *145*
Klevecz, R. R., 25, 29, 33-34, *41-42*
Klinger, I., 162, 164, *173*
Klug, A., 122, *126*
Knecht, M. E., 170, *173*
Knight, J., 167, *174*
Kobayashi, Y., 54, *75*
Koerner, D., 114, *130*
Koga, M., 63, *74*, 82, *103*
Kohn, H. I., 27, *29*, 35, *41*
Koide, T. J., 57, *76*
Kolitsky, M. A., 168, *174*
Kolodny, E. H., 149, *157*, 171, *173*
Koprowski, H., 57, *74*, 211, *213*
Kornberg, A., 19, 21, *29, 31*
Kornberg, R. D., 109, *128*
Korner, A., 141, *144*
Kornfeld, S., 154, *158*
Kostraba, N. C., 88, 98-99, *104*, 115-116, 123, *128*
Kraemer, P. M., 36, *42*, 151, *158*
Krause, M. D., 212, *214*
Kruh, J., 121, *127*

Kruse, P. F. Jr., 11, *15*, 163, *173*, 181, *187*
Kudlow, J. E., 141, *144*, 181, *187*, 197, *198*
Kuempel, P. L., 24, *30*
Kufe, D., 209, *214*

L

Labows, J., 65, *75*
Lafarge, C., 193, *198*
Laine, R., 149, *158*
Lajtha, L. G., 175, *188*
Lake, R. S., 39, *42*
Lallier, R., 150, *157*
Lambert, W. C., 18, *29-30*
Lamerton, L. F., 4, 10, *15*, 50, *51*
Langan, T. A., 33, *41*
Lapeyre, J., 114, *126*
Lark, K. G., 14, *15*, 21, 24, *29*, 39, *42*, 79, *104*
Larsson, A., 22, *29*
Laskey, R. A., 6, *15*
Laurence, E. B., 34, *41*, 167, 170, *172-173*
Lavender, K., 196, *198*
Laude, J. P., 44, 47, *51*
Lazar, G. K., 7, *16*, 56, 77, 82, *106*
Lebeau, M., 155, *158*
Lee, J. C. K., 167, *173*
Lee, K., 58, *75*, 168, *173*
Lee-Huang, S., 142, *145*
Leighton, J. T., 110, *128*
Leon, M. A., 56, *76*
Leong, G. F., 167, *173*
Lerner, A. B., 34, *42*
Lerner, R. A., 47, *52*
Lesher, S., 27, *29*, 35, *41*
Lesser, B., 58, *75*
Le Stourgeon, W. M., 121, *128*

Levene, C. I., 164-165, *172*
Levi-Montalcini, R., 165, *173*
Levine, E. M., 185, *188*
Levine, S., 165-166, *173*
Levinson, B. B., 139-140, *145*
Levinson, W., 209, *214*
Levinthal, C., 54, *75*
Levitt, J., 56, *73*
Levy, R., 120-121, *128*
Levy, S., 114, 120-121, *128*
Ley, K. D., 19, *29*, 57, 77, 179, *188*
Liao, S., 87, *104*
Lieberman, I., 22, *28*, 32, *42*, 44, 50,
    52, 57-58, 60, 63, 69, *74-77*, 81-
    82, 101, *103-104, 106*, 142, *145*,
    168, *174*, 181, *187*
Lin, A. H., 87, *104*
Lin, J., 116, *130*
Lin, J. C., 212, *214*
Lindahl, G., 210, *214*
Lindsay, V. J., 69, *75*
Lipkin, G., 170, *173*
Lipkin, M., 13, *15, 29*, 35, *42*
Lipton, A., 162, 164-166, *173*
Liskay, R. M., 48, *52*
Littau, V. C., 109, *126*
Litwack, G., 62, 64, *77*
Lockwood, D. H., 57, 69, *75-76*
Lodish, H. F., 71, *74*, 100, *103*
Loeb, L. A., 205, *214*
Loeb, J. E., 116, *128*
Lowenstein, W. R., 171, *173*
Lopez, C., 67-68, *74*
Lopez-Saez, J. F., 20, *29*
Luwick, T. M., 89, *102*
Lundeen, D. E., 56, *76*
Lurquin, P. F., 94-95, 97, *104-106*

M

MacGillivrary, A. J., 87-88, *104*, 107-
    108, 111-113, *128-129*

Macieira-Coelho, A., 50, *52*, 56, *75*
MacLeod, C. M., 2, *15*
MacPherson, I., 152, *157*
Maizel, A., 137-138, *145*, 185, *188*
Majumdar, C., 63, *76*, 142, *145*
Malaise, E., 27, *29*, 50, *51*
Malamud, D., 3, 13, *15*, 58, *76*, 197,
    198
Malloy, G. R., 100, *103*
Malpoix, P., 26, *31*
Malt, R. A., 58, *76*, 197, *198*
Mamont, P., 183, *187*
Maniatis, G. M., 63, *76*, 82, *104*
Mankovitz, R., 79, *106*
Manson, L. A., 27, *28*, 35, *41*
Marcus, P. I., 37, *42*
Marks, D., 33, *42*
Marks, D. B., 26, *30*, 47, *52*
Marks, P. A., 63, *76*, 82, *104*, 115,
    128
Marsh, W. H., 58, *74*
Marti, A., 165, *172*
Martin, D., Jr., 47, *52*
Martin, G. M., 9, *15*
Martin, L., 120, *128*
Martin, M. A., 210, *214*
Martinez-Palomo, A., 148, *158*
Marton, L. J., 69, *75*
Marushige, K., 84, *86-87, 103-104,*
    109, 113, 116, *126, 128*
Maruta, H., 122, *128*
Maryanka, D., 87, *104*
Masker, W. E., 23, *30*
Massol, N., 155, *158*
Masui, H., 58, *76*
Mathias, A. P., 116, *127*
Matthews, H. R., 33, *41*
Mauck, J. C., 63, *76*, 92, *104*
Mauel, J., 165-166, *173*
Maul, G., 186, *188*
Mayfield, J. E., 88, *104*
Mayhew, E., 36, *42*
Mayzel, W., 1, *15*

McCarthy, B. J., 70-71, *74*, 98-99, 101, *103*
McCarty, M., 2, *15*
McClure, M. D., 108, 113, *128*
McCulloch, E. A., 166, *174*
McFarland, V. W., 149, *157*
McGhee, J. D., 23, *29*
McGuire, J. S., 34, *42*
Means, A. R., 100, *104*, 195-196, *199*
Medeiros, E., 210, *214*
Meiss, H. K., 48, *51*, 79-80, *103, 106*, 197, *199*
Meister, A., 153, *158*
Mendelsohn, J., 83, *105*, 154, *158*
Merriam, R. W., 137, *145*
Mertens, J. G., 181, *187*
Messner, H. A., 166, *174*
Metcalf, D., 165-166, *173*
Metha, S., 186, *188*
Meza, I., 71, *74*
Micali, A., 25, *30*, 60, *76*
Miedema, E., 11, *15*, 163, *173*
Mihm, M. C., 206, *213*
Miller, O. H., 58, *75*
Miller, O. N., 168, *173*
Millis, A. J. T., 34, *42*
Mironescu, S., 63, *74*, 164, *172*
Mirsky, A. E., 194, *198*
Mitchell, R. A., 168, *174*
Mitchell, W. M., 90, 94, *105*, 121, *129*
Mitchison, J. M., 14, *16*
Miyagi, M., 88, *105*
Miyakawa, N., 116, *128*
Mizuno, D., 122, *128*
Mohla, S., 196, *198*
Monjardino, J. P. P. V., 111, *129*
Monod, J., 78, *104*
Mons, M., 119, 121, *130*
Moolten, F., 167, *172*
Moore, G. P. M., 137, *144*
Moore, S., 108, *127*

Moorhead, P. S., 24, *30*
Mora, P. T., 149, *157*
Mordoh, J., 20, *29*
Morishima, A., 24, *30*
Morley, A., 35, *43*
Morris, H. P., 35, *42*
Morris, T. W., 169, *173*
Moscovici, G., 113, 119, 121, *130*
Moses, R. E., 20, *30*
Moudrianakis, E. N., 95, *102*
Muchmore, J., 60, *77*
Mueller, G. C., 17, 20, *30*, 47, *52*, 63, 77, 82, *106*, 142, *147*, 152, *157*
Mueller, G. M., 87, *105*
Mulcahy, H. L., 20, *30*
Murphy, E. C., Jr., 117, 124, *129*

N

Nations, C., 121, *128*
Nervi, C., 203-204, *213*
Ng, S., 124, *129*
Nias, A. H. W., 18, *30*
Nicolini, C., 21, *30*, 94-97, *102, 104*, 124, *129*, 137-138, *145*, 185, *188*, 212, *214*
Nicolson, G. L., 149, *158*
Niessing, J., 100, *104*
Nigam, V. N., 150, *157*
Noble, A., 194, *199*
Nola, E., 195, *199*
Nomura, M., 122, *130*
Nonoyama, M., 23, *29*
Noonan, K. D., 71, *76*, 148-149, *157, 159*
Nordling, S., 57, *77*, 165, *174*
Norrby, K., 11, *16*
North, A. B., 211, *213*
Norwood, T. H., 9, *15*
Novakova, V., 194, *199*
Nova, A. M., 63-66, *76*, 83, 89-90, *104*, 112, *129*, 178, *188*, 192, *199*

Nowell, P., 56, *76*
Nowinski, R. C., 210, *214*
Nuret, P., 101, *103*
Nuzzo, F., 22, *30*
Nygaard, O., 60, *76*

O

Oakman, N. J., 61, *73*
Ochoa, S., 142, *145*
O'Conner, A., 12, *15*, 27, *28*, 35, *41*
Oey, J., 67, *76*, 163, *173*
Ohkita, T., 12, *15*, 27, *28*, 35, *41*
Ohlenbusch, H., 84, 86, *103*
Okada, S., 45, 47, 50, *51*
Olivera, B., 84, 86, *103*
O'Malley, B. W., 90, 94, 100, *104-
    105*, 121-122, *129*, 195-196, *199*
Omine, M., 69, *75*
Ono, T., 140, *145*
Onoda T., 37, *43*
Oppenheimer, J. H., 114, *130*
Ota, K., 12, *13*, 27, *28*, 35, *41*
Ove, P., 44, 50, *52*, 57, 63, *75*, 81,
    104
Oyanguren, C., 82, *105*
Ozaki, H., *129*

P

Pagano, J. S., 24, *29*
Paik, W. K., 26, *30*, 33, *42*, 47, *52*,
    110, *129*
Painter, R. B., 24, *30*
Paoluzi, R., 203-204, *213*
Pappenheimer, A. M., Jr., 143, *144*
Pardee, A. B., 46, 49, *51-52*, 83, *103*,
    146-147, 149-156, *157-158*, 177,
    179, 181-182, *187, 188*
Parker, C. W., 46, *52*
Pastan, I., 67, *75-76*, 112, *129*

Pasternak, C. A., 152, *158*
Patterson, B. D., 110, *129*
Paul, D., 67, 77, 162, 164, *173*
Paul, J., 85, 87-88, *104*, 107-108,
    111-113, 115-116, *127-129*
Pawelek, J., 34, *42*
Pearson, G. D., 24, *30*
Pearson, W. R., 108, 114, *127*
Pedersen, T., 45, *52*
Pedrini, A. M., 22, *30*
Pegg, A. O., 69, *76*
Pegoraro, L., 60-61, *76*
Pelc, S. R., 2, *15*
Pendergrass, W. R., 9, *15*
Penman, S., 38, *41*, 101, *102*, 197,
    198
Penon, P., 89, *105*
Perez, A. G., 47, *51*
Perlman, R., 112, *129*
Perretta, M., 82, *105*
Perrin, L., 58, *76*
Perry, R. P., 49, *52*, 84, *105*, 140,
    145
Perry, S., 69, *75*
Petersen, D. F., 32-33, 35, *42*
Petersen, R. O., 44-45, 47, *51*, 116,
    130
Peterson, J. A., 152, *158*
Philipson, L., 50, *52*
Phillips, C., 110, *128*
Philpott, G. W., 46, *52*
Pickart, L., 165, *173*
Pictet, R. L., 165-166, 169, *173*
Pierson, R. W., Jr., 155, *158*, 166,
    173
Pileri, A., 12-13, *15*, 202, *213*
Pious, D. A., 34, *42*
Platz, R. D., 116, *129*
Pogo, A. O., 82, 88, *105*, 110-111,
    120, *129*
Pogo, B. G. T., 82, 88, *105*, 110-111,
    120, *129*
Pogell, B. M., 93, *105*

Połacow, J., 94, *105*
Pollack, R., 67, *76*, 163, *173*
Pollister, A. W., 113, *128*
Ponten, J., 11, 13, *16*, 50, *52*, 56-57, 75-76, 146-147, 150, 163, *173*
Poste, G., 150, *158*
Potter, V. R., 141, *145*
Powell, A. E., 56, *76*
Prescott, D. M., 23-24, 26, *28, 30,* 37-38, *42*, 136, *145*
Price, G. B., 166, *174*
Pringle, J. R., 14, 15, 79, *104*
Puca, G. A., 195, *199*

Q

Quastler, H., 4, *16*
Quintrell, N., 210, *214*

R

Rachmeler, M., 66, *74*
Radda, G. K., 94, *104*
Radley, J. M., 33, *42*, 192, *199*
Raff, R. A., 140, *145*
Raick, A. N., 58, *76*
Raina, A., 68-69, *76*
Rainey, C., 117, *129*
Rajewsky, M. F., 212, *213*
Ramos, J., 27, *30*
Rao, P. N., 20, *30*, 34, *42*
Raska, K., Jr., 56, 67, *77*
Rasmussen, R. E., 24, *30*
Ratliff, R. L., 47-48, *52*
Reddan, J. R., 180, *187*
Reddy, V. N., 180, *187*
Reeck, G. R., 117, *129*
Reed, W. B., 208, *213*
Reeder, 87, *105*
Reeve, P., 150, *158*
Reid, B. J., 14, *15*, 79, *104*

Rejman, E., 70, *74*
Remington, J. A., 34, *42*
Remo, R. A., 22, *28*, 61, *74*
Renger, H. C., 67, *73*
Ricard, J., 89, *105*
Richards, C., 58, *74*
Richardson, C. C., 20, *30*
Richter, G. W., 58, *73*, 178, *187*
Richter, K. H., 114, 116, *129*
Rifkind, R. A., 63, *76*, 82, *104*, 115, *128*
Rigler, R., 93-95, *105*
Ringertz, N. R., 93-95, 98, *103, 105,* 136-137, *144-145*, 185, *187*
Ristow, H. J., 164-166, *172*
Robbins, E., 25, *28, 30*, 37, *42*, 47, 50, *51*, 60, *76*, 113, *126*
Robbins, P. W., 149, 151, *159*
Robbins, S. L., 190, *199*
Robertson, J. S., 27, *29*
Robinson, H., 48, *52*
Rogentine, G. N., Jr., 18, *28*
Rogers, A. W., 3, *16*
Rogue, A., 58, *74*
Roos, B. A., 83, *105*
Roscoe, D. H., 48, *52*
Rose, N. R., 113, *126*, 137, *144*
Rosenberg, S. A., 120-121, *128*
Rosenfeld, M. G., 83, *105*
Rosenstock, L., 58, *74*
Roth, G. S., 180, *187*
Rothstein, A., 47, *51*
Rovera, G., 49-50, *51-52*, 55, 72, *73-74*, 82-83, 89-91, *103, 105*, 109, 111, 118, 120, 124, *126, 129*, 131-132, 138, *144-145*, 154, *158*, 177, 181, 184, 186, *187-188*
Rozengurt, E., 153-154, 156, *157*
Rubin, A. O., 82, *103*
Rubin, H., 57, *76*, 143, *144*, 152, 154, *158* 163, *173-174*
Ruddon, R. W., 56, *76*, 114, 117, *129*, 134, *145*, 212, *214*

Rudland, P. S., 67, *77*
Ruoslahti, E., 57, *77*, 165, *174*
Rusch, H. P., 32, *41*, 60, *76*, 121, *128*
Rusconi, M., 1, *16*
Russell, D. H., 68-69, *75-76*
Russell, T. R., 67, *76*
Russev, G., 25, *31*
Rutter, W. J., 165-166, 169, *173*
Ryan, W. L., 67, *75*

S

Sachs, L., 148-149, *158*, 170, *174*
Sage, N., 82, *105*
Saito, M., 21, *30*
Salas, J., 56, *76*
Salb, J. M., 37, *42*
Salser, W., 70, *76*
Salzman, N. P., 39, *42*
Sambrook, J., 37, *42*, 211, *213*
Sams, B. F., 193, *199*
Sander, G., 46, *52*, 154, *158*, 177, 179, 181-182, *188*
Sandritter, W., 191, 194, *198-199*
Sankaran, L., 93, *105*
Sarkar, N. H., 210, *214*
Sarna, G. P., 69, *75*
Sasaki, T., 35, *42*, 62, 64, *77*
Sato, S., 21, *30*
Sauer, G., 56, *77*
Sauerbier, W., 100, *104*
Saunders, E. H., 58, *75*
Saunders, G. F., 87, *106*
Sawicki, S. G., 131, *145*
Scharff, M. D., 25, *28*, 37, *42*, 47-50, *51*, 113, *126*
Schauder, P., 117, *126*
Scheffler, I., 20, *29*
Scheffler, I. E., 80, *105*
Scher, C. D., 166, *173*

Scher, W., 56, *74*
Schekman, R., 21, *31*
Schimke, R. T., 113, *127*
Schizuya, H., 20, *30*
Schlueter, G., 194, *199*
Schlom, J., 209, *213*
Schnebli, H. P., 135, *145*, 169, *174*
Schneyer, C. A., 192, *199*
Schochetman, G., 140, *145*
Schrader, W. T., 122, *129*
Schrock, T., 167, *172*
Schroeder, J. L., 67, *75*
Schulter, G., 191, *198*
Schweiger, M., 100, *104*
Schweppe, J. S., 134, *145*
Scomazzoni, G., 191, *199*
Sefton, B. M., 154, *158*
Seifert, W., 67, *77*
Sekeris, C. E., 100, *104*, 114, 116, *129*
Seligy, V. L., 94-95, *105-106*
Sellers, L., 47, *51*
Selvig, S. E., 140, *145*
Settineri, D., 121, *126*
Shaeffer, J. R., 47, 49, *52*
Sharma, V. K., 170, *173*
Shearer, W. T., 46, *52*
Sheehy, P. F., 20, *30*
Shelton, K., 117, *129*
Shepherd, J. H., 117, 124, *129*
Sheppard, J. R., 36, *41*, 66-67, *73*, *77*, 151, *157*
Sherman, M. R., 196, *199*
Sherlock, P., 27, *29*, 35, *42*
Sherman, F. G., 4, *16*
Shields, R., 183, *187*
Shinitzky, M., 149, *158*
Shodell, M., 155, *158*, 165-166, *174*
Short, J., 58, 69, *74*, *77*, 168, *174*
Sibatani, A., 193, *198*
Sica, V., 195, *199*
Siimes, M., 68, *76*

Simard, A., 170, *174*
Siminovitch, L., 79, *106*
Simmons, T., 50, *52*
Simpson, R. T., 86, 93-94, *105*, 107, 113-114, 117, 120-121, 124, *128-129*, 132, *145*
Sisken, J. E., 33, *42*
Skinner, A. M., 56, *73*, 154, *158*
Slater, I., 140, *145*
Slater, D. W., 140, *145*
Smart, J. E., 124, *129*
Smellie, R. M. S., 154, *156*, 183, *187*
Smets, L. A., 95, *105*, 149, *156*, 177, 184, *188*, 211, *214*
Smith, B. M., 80, *105*
Smith, D. W., 20, *30*
Smith, E. L., 108, 110, *127-128*
Smith, J. A., 120, *129*
Smith, H. S., 210, *214*
Snyder, S. H., 68-69, *75-76*
Sober, H. A., 94, *105*, 114, 117, *128-129*
Soeiro, R., 141, *145*
Sommer, K. R., 110, *128*
Sören, L., 178, *188*
Spadari, S., 20, *30*
Speight, V. A., 22, *29*
Spelsberg, T. C., 90, 94, 101, *104-106*, 115-116, 119-122, *126-127*, *129-130*, 155, *157*, 195-196, *198-199*
Spiegelman, S., 209, *213-214*
Spinelli, G., 121, *126*
Sporn, M. B., 85-87, *103*, 110, 113, 116, *127*
Sprague, C. A., 9, *15*
Springgate, C. F., 205, *214*
Srivastava, B. I. S., 133, *145*
Stadler, J. K., 36, *42*
Stambrook, P. J., 23, *30*
Stanners, C. P., 121, *126*, 141, *144*, 181, *187*, 197, *198*

Stastny, M., 141, *144*
Stathakos, D., 166, *173*
Steel, G. G., 12, *16*, 202, 206, *213*, *214*
Steggles, A. W., 122, *129*, 195-196, *199*
Stein, G., 18, 26, *30*, 37-38, *41-42*, 66, *73*, 77, 82, *105*, 108, 113-114, 117-122, 124, *126*, 131, 135, *145*, 180, 183, *187*, 212, *214*
Stein, W. H., 108, *127*
Steinberg, W., 54, *75*
Stellwagen, R. H., 108-110, 113, 120, *130*
Stellwagen, R. H., 108-110, 113, 120, *130*
Stern, H., 194, *198*
Steward, D. L., 47, 49, *52*
Stock, J. J., 110, *128*
Stockdale, F. E., 57, *75*
Stoddard, S. K., 58, *76*
Stoker, M. G. P., 146, *159*, 163, 167, 171, *172*, *174*
Stollar, B. D., 110, *126*
Stryckmans, P., 27, *30*
Stubblefield, E., 23-24, *30*, 39, *42*, 47, *52*
Studzinski, G. P., 18, *29-30*, 121, *126*, 197, *199*, 211-212, *213*
Sudweeks, A. D., 142, *145*
Sueoka, N., 54, *73*
Sugimura, T., 21, *30*
Summers, W. P., 87, *105*
Sun, S., 58, *75*, 168, *173*
Sung, M. T., 111, *130*
Surks, M. I., 114, *130*
Swaffield, M., 167, *172*
Swaneck, G. E., 117, *130*
Swartz, F., 193, *199*
Swern, D., 65, *75*
Szirmai, J. A., 190, *199*
Szirmal, J. A., 190, *199*

T

Tack, L. O., 113, *126*
Taft, D. O., 196, *199*
Tait, R. C., 20, *30*
Takahashi, H., 37, *43*
Takai, S., 60, *77*
Talmadge, K. W., 149, *159*
Tamm, I., 24, *29*
Tan, C. H., 88, *105*
Tanaka, A., 23, *29*
Tanaka, M., 21, *30*
Tarbutt, R. G., 50, *51*
Tata, J. R., 73, *77*, 82, 85, *104-105*,
    197, *199*, 212, *214*
Taylor, C. W., 212, *214*
Taylor, D. M., 53, 58, *77*, 82, *105-*
    106
Taylor, J. H., 24, *30-31*, 38, *42*
Taylor, R. L., 69, *76*
Teather, C., 148, *158*
Teissere, M., 89, *105*
Telaranta, T., 69, *76*
Temin, H. M., 53, 57, 72, *74, 77*,
    155, *158*, 165-166, *172-173*, 184,
    188
Teng, C. S., 85, 89, *105*, 120, *130*
Terasima, T., 18, 27, *31*, 35, *42*, 45,
    47, 50, *52*
Terayama, H., 88, *102*
Terskikh, V. V., 7-8, *15*, 55, *74*, 177,
    187
Thackrah, T., 114, *127*
Thaler, M. M., 89, *105*, 165, *173*
Thomson, J. A., 68, *73*, 89, *103*
Thomas, J. D., 109, *128*
Thomson, J. A., 133, *144*
Thompson, L., 79, *106*
Thrall, C. L., 113, *130*
Thrash, C. R., 155, *157*
Threlfall, G., 53, 58, *77*, 82, 87-88,
    104-106, 107-108, 111-113, *128*
Till, A. R., 50, *51*

Till, J. E., 79, *106*, 166, *174*
Tobey, R. A., 19, *29*, 32-33, 35-36,
    42, 47-48, *52*, 57, 77, 151, *158*,
    179, *188*
Todaro, G. J., 7, *16*, 56, *77*, 82, *106*,
    162, 164, *173*, 182, *188*
Toft, D., 153, *159*
Tolmach, L. J., 18, 27, *31*, 35, *42*,
    50, *52*
Tomaszewski, M., 70, *74*
Tomatis, L., 209, *214*
Tomkins, G. M., 47, *52*, 139-140,
    145, 183, *187*
Toniolo, D., 79, *106*, 197, *199*
Topper, Y. J., 57, *75*
Tormey, D. C., 63, *77*
Touraine, F., 67-68, *74*
Touraine, J., 67-68, *74*
Traub, P., 122, *130*
Troll, W., 89, *104*
Trowbridge, I. S., 150, *159*
Trudel, M., 150, *157*
Tsai, A., 24, *29*
Tsai, M., 87, *106*
Tsai, R. L., 92, *106*
Tsanev, R., 25, *31*
Tsuboi, A., 121, *130, 145*
Tsuchiya, T., 122, *128*
Tsukada, K., 63, *76, 106*, 142, *145*
Tuan, D., 109, *126*
Tubiana, M., 18, 27, *29*, 50, *51*
Turkington, R. W., 57, *77*, 212, *213*
Turner, G. N., 24, *29*

U

Ui, H., 82, *106*
Uthne, K., 166, *172*

V

Vaheri, A., 57, *77*, 165, *174*
Valenzuela, A., 82, *105*

van Beek, W. P., 149, *156*
Van den Berg, K. J., 154-155, *159*
Van Eupen, O., 116, *127*
Van Potter, V. R., 60, *75*
Varga, J. M., 34, *42*
Varnus, H. E., 209-210, *214*
Vassort, F., 50, *51*
Veda, K., 114, *128*
Vendrely, C., 5, *15*
Vendrely, R., 5, *15*
Venoyama, K., 140, *145*
Verly, W. E., 170, *174*
Vertes, M., 120, *129*
Vesser, J., 164-166, *172*
Vidali, G., 33, *42*, 114, 119, *128,*
  130, 137, *144*
Villee, C. A., 89, *105*
Virolainen, M., 57, *77*
Vogel, A., 67, *76*, 163, *173*
Vogt, M., 56, *74*
von Hippel, P. H., 23, *29*

W

Wagner, T., 94, *106*
Wakabayashi, K., 212, *214*
Wake, S. K., 108, 114, *127*
Wakonig-Vaartaja, T., 20, *30*
Walker, I. O., 94, *104*
Walter, S., 165-166, *173*
Walters, R. A., 47-48, *52*
Wang, J. L., 180, *187*
Wang, T. Y., 88, 98-99, *104*, 115-
  116, 123, *128, 130*
Warren, J. C., 85, 88-89, *102*
Warren, L., 152, *159*
Waymouth, C., 161-162, *174*
Webb, T. E., 141, *145*
Weber, M. J., 186, *188*
Weber, J. J., 147, *159*
Wechsler, J. A., 19, *29*
Weil, R. L., 170, *173*

Weisenthal, L. M., 56, *76*, 134, *145,*
  212, *214*
Weiser, R. S., 117, 124, *129*
Weiss, R. A., 209, *214*
Weissbach, A., 20, *30*
Weissman, G., 89, *104*
Wells, J. R. E., 110, *126*
Westermark, B., 13, *16*, 57, *76*, 163,
  174
Whalen, R. G., 71, *73*
Wheatley, D. N., 33, *43*
Whelley, S. M., 142-143, *145*
White, A., 56, *77*
Whitmore, G. F., 79, *106*
Whittle, W., 11, *15*, 163, *173*
Wickner, W., 21, *31*
Wickus, G. G., 149, *159*
Widholm, J., 84, 86, *103*
Widnell, C. C., 82, *104*
Wiebel, F., 56, *77*, 143, *145*, 183,
  188, 202, *213*
Wied, G. L., 197, *198*
Wigglesworth, N. M., 80, *105*
Wilhelm, J. A., 86, *106*
Wilkes, E., 33, *42*
Williams, A. F., 110, *126*
Williams, R. E., 94-95, *106*
Williams-Ashman, H. G., 69, *76*
Willingham, M. C., 67, *76*
Wilson, E. M., 90, 94, *105*, 121, *129*
Wilson, P. A., 50, *51*
Wilson, J. R., 180, *187*
Wilson, W. L., 180, *187*
Wilt, F. H., 140, *145*
Winick, M., 194, *199*
Winn, R., 20, *30*
Wolf, B. A., 151, *159*
Wostenholme, G. E. W., 167, *174*
Wray, W., 121, *128*
Wright, J. A., 79, *106*
Wright, N., 35, *43*
Wright, W. E., 37, *43*, 211, *214*
Wu, F. C., 114, *130*, 149, *159*

Y

Yaoi, Y., 37, *43*
Yasukawa, M., 45, 47, *52*
Yeh, J., 170, *174*
Yeoman, L. C., 212, *214*
Yoshikura, H., 56, 77
Young, K. E., 114, *126*, 212, *213*
Younkin, L. H., 178, *188*

Z

Zampetti-Bosseler, F., 26, *31*
Zardi, L., 63, 69, *75*, 77, 116, *130*, 212, *214*
Zatz, M. M., 56, 77
Zemel, R., 58, 77, 168, *174*
Zetterberg, A., 95, *106*, 137, *144*
Ziegler, J. L., 203-204, *213*
Zimmerman, J. E., Jr., 56, 67, 77
Ziparo, E., 203-204, *213*
Zweig, M., 141, *145*

SUBJECT INDEX

A

Acetabularia, 189
Acridine orange, 92-95, 211
ACTH, 58
Actinomycin D, 44, 45, 49, 62, 71,
        81, 83, 84, 93, 124, 125,
        131, 132
S-Adenosyl-L-methionine, 68
Adenovirus, 56
Adenyl cyclase, 33
Poly-ADP-ribose, 25, 114
Adrenal glands, 58
Albumin, 63, 142, 143, 164
    depletion, 58
Aldosterone, 117
Allium cepa, 20
2-Amino-isobutyric acid, 154, 179
Aminonucleoside, 211
Amnion cells, 165
Amoeba, 136
α-Amylase, 62, 64, 83

Anchorage dependence, 146
Androgen(s), 69, 120
Antibodies, 46, 47
Antibody- forming cells, 13
Ataxia telangiectasia, 207
5-Azacytidine, 132
Azathioprine, 197

B

Bacillus subtilis, 79
Bacteria, 14, 19, 20, 21, 54
BHK cells, 67, 79, 119, 120, 134,
        148, 155, 163, 165, 166
Bronchus, 13, 27
    carcinoma, 13, 27
Burkitt lymphoma, 204
Bone marrow, 2, 5
Brain, 85, 88, 212
Bromodeoxyuridine, 211

C

Carp, 110
Carcinomas
    epidermoid, 207
Carcinomas of head
    squamous cell, 204
Cartilage, 58
Catalase, 140
Cd^{++}, 57
    cell fusion, 57
    loss, 10-12
Centrioles, 25, 60
Chalones, 34, 47, 169, 170
Chinese hamster cells, 23, 24, 32-34,
    36, 38, 153, 154, 179,
    182
Chromatin, 17, 23, 38, 45, 68, 85-88,
    96-99, 107, 109, 115,
    117, 121, 122, 124, 135,
    194-196, 212
    reconstitution, 39, 123
    structure, 92, 132
    template activity, 38, 39, 49,
        84, 88, 90, 91, 93, 96,
        101, 111, 112, 118, 122,
        123, 183, 184, 196
    thermal stability, 94, 98
Chromosomal proteins, 25, 39
Chromosome, 23, 24, 26, 38, 93, 94,
    96-98, 124
Colon
    carcinoma, 27
    epithelial cells, 13, 35
Concanavalin A, 56, 137, 148, 150,
    154, 155, 180, 185
Conditioned medium, 57
Contact inhibition, 146, 147, 171
Cortisol, 117
Croton oil, 58
Cyclic AMP, 34, 66-68, 112, 133,
    153, 163

Cyclic GMP, 67, 68
Cytochalasin B, 37, 211
Cycloheximide, 111, 138, 141, 155
Cycloleucine, 154, 182

D

dCMP Deaminase, 47
Density-dependent inhibition, 67,
    146, 147
2-Deoxyglucose, 154, 182
Deoxynucleotides, 21-23, 26, 47, 48,
    61
5-a-Dihydrotestosterone, 58
1-a,25-Dihydroxycholecalciferol, 153
7,12-Dimethylbenz(A)anthacene,
    209
Diphtheria toxin, 143
DNA, 2-5, 8, 10, 24, 85
    polymerase, 19-21, 61, 79, 114,
        180, 205
    satellite, 87
    sequences, 99
    synthesis, 4-8, 12-14, 19-26,
        39, 40, 44-46, 54, 60, 61,
        63, 65, 67, 71, 72, 79,
        81, 90, 91, 98, 123, 177,
        195, 208
DNA-binding protein, 23
DNase, 132
DNA/RNA hybridization, 98
γDNA, 87
Drosophila, 111
Duodenal crypt cells, 13, 27

E

E. coli, 80, 86-88, 90, 101, 142, 210
E. coli RNA,
    polymerase, 91

Eggs, 6, 10, 23
Embryo cells, 13, 27, 35, 37, 50
Endometrium,
    carcinoma, 13
Epidermal growth factor, 57, 124,
        141, 165
Epidermis, 2, 5, 6, 34, 165, 177
Epstein-Barr herpesvirus, 23
Erythroblasts, 50
Erythrocyte(s), 6, 7, 85, 87, 94, 95,
        110, 113, 123, 136, 185,
        194
    nuclei, 94, 137
Erthyropoietin, 58, 82
Esophageal,
    carcinoma, 27
    epithelium, 27
Estradiol, 88, 89, 100, 120, 195
Estrogens, 7, 55, 58, 63, 69, 82, 88,
        94, 101, 120, 121, 143,
        153, 154, 156, 183, 195,
        196
Ethidium bromide, 93, 95, 97, 124
Ethionine, 58
Ethylphenylpropiolate, 58
Euplotes, 26

F

FGF, 165
Fibroblasts, 47, 50, 57, 89, 120, 154,
        155, 165, 166, 181, 183,
        197
    human diploid, 4, 13, 24, 27,
        35, 49, 50, 66, 71, 82,
        83, 90, 92, 94-96, 101,
        109, 111, 118, 120-122,
        131, 134, 137, 138, 143,
        153, 154, 163-165, 179,
        180, 182, 183, 185, 212
p-Fluorophenylalanine, 33

Folic acid, 58, 68, 82, 89, 133
Friend leukemia, 56

G

G_0, 7, 18, 179, 182
G_0 cells, 8-10, 12-14, 50, 53-55, 60,
        70, 72, 80, 81, 88, 90,
        98, 131, 139, 147, 151,
        153, 175, 177, 179, 200,
        202
G_1, 3-5, 8, 9, 14, 18-20, 25, 45-47
G_1 cells, 9, 44-47, 49, 50, 175, 179,
        181
G_2, 3-5, 7, 8, 13, 14, 18-20, 22, 25,
        28, 32, 34, 37, 40, 45,
        53, 60, 194, 196
    arrest, 34
    length, 34
G_2 cells, 12, 33
    arrested, 40
Gangliosides, 149
Genes, 65, 99, 100, 139
    activity, 98, 116, 142
    expression, 38, 70, 80, 107,
        108, 111, 112, 115, 119
    methylation, 111
Glia-like cells, 13, 163
Glioma cells, 13
Glucagon, 58, 168
Glycolipids, 148-152
Glycoproteins, 149
Glycosidases, 148
Growth factors, 160, 167
Growth fraction, 10-12, 201, 203,
        204, 206
Growth hormone, 58

H

Heart, 190, 191, 194

HeLa cells, 7, 13, 20, 21, 27, 35, 45,
        50, 119, 121, 122, 135-
        137, 185
Heparin, 36, 168
Heparin sulfate, 151
Hepatocytes (see also Liver), 13, 142,
        143, 165, 177, 180
Hepatoma, 13, 35, 167, 212
Herpes simplex virus, 150
Heterochromatin, 186
Heterokaryons, 135
High-protein diet, 58
Histones, 17, 25, 26, 39, 48, 86, 107-
        109, 112-114, 122, 124
    acetylated, 110, 111
    methylated, 110
    phosphorylated, 33, 46, 47,
        110, 111
Histone mRNA, 47
Hydra attenuata, 40
Hydrocortisone, 165
Hydroxyurea, 177
Hyperplasia, 190-192, 195, 196
Hypertrophy, 190, 191, 193-197

                            I

Immunosuppressive agents, 196-197
Indole-3-acetic acid, 89
Inhibition,
    density-dependent, 67, 146,
        147
Insulin, 57, 117, 165, 166
Intestinal,
    crypts, 32
Interphase, 1, 2, 38
1-Phenyl-2-Isopropylaminoethanol,
        91, 118
Isoproterenol, 7, 33, 55, 58-65, 82,
        83, 89-91, 112, 117, 120,
        124, 131, 133, 143, 178,
        180, 191, 192

                            K

Kidney, 34, 44, 50, 58, 68, 82, 85,
        89, 117, 133, 178

                            L

L cells, 13, 25, 27, 35, 45, 50, 140,
        166, 181
Lactation, 89, 120
Lead, 178
Lead acetate, 58
Lectins, 56, 149
Lens culinaris, 89
Leukemia, 13
Leukocytes,
    polymorphonuclear, 2, 6
Liver, 58, 85, 88, 89, 94, 99, 108,
        115, 120, 121, 155, 193,
        194, 212
    regenerating, 7, 22, 35, 40, 50,
        55, 58, 60, 61, 63, 68,
        69, 71, 81, 82, 88, 98,
        99, 101, 111, 112, 141,
        167
Lymphnodes, 177
Lymphocytes, 7, 22, 34, 35, 46, 55,
        63, 67, 68, 82, 83, 88,
        89, 93-96, 111, 120, 121,
        135, 137, 141, 142, 152,
        154, 178, 180, 185, 212
Lymphoid cells (see also Cells),
    human, 18, 34, 23
Lymphosarcoma, 13

                            M

Macrophage, 165, 186,
Mammary gland, 13, 27, 50, 58, 89,
        120, 210
Melanocytes, 47, 186

Melanocyte-stimulating hormone, 34
Melanoma, 206
"Melting protein," 23
Membranes, 36, 37, 65, 146, 147,
      149, 151, 152, 184
   function, 153
Micrococcus lysodeikticus, 86
Microfilaments, 37
Microtubules, 35
Microtubular proteins, 33
Mitosis, 1-6, 8, 13, 14, 18, 22, 32-38,
      40, 50, 66, 114, 194, 197
   length, 34
Mn^{++}, 57
Mutants,
   temperature-sensitive, 19, 48,
      79, 80, 197

N

N-Acetylgalactosaminyl-transferase,
   149
$NaIO_4$, 56
Nephrectomy, 58
Nerve growth factor, 165
Neuraminidase, 57, 165
Neurons, 2,6,7,165
Neurospora crassa, 110
Newcastle disease virus, 150
NIL 8 cells, 150
N-methyl-N'-nitro-N-nitroso-guani-
   dine, 48
N,N-dimethyl-p-(m-tolyazo)-aniline,
   90, 119
Nonhistone chromosomal proteins,
      17, 25, 26, 39, 85, 107-
      109, 113-118, 120, 121,
      123, 125, 132, 133, 137-
      139, 143, 181, 185, 186,
      212
   acetylation, 134
   phosphorylation, 119, 134

   synthesis, 37, 65, 66, 72
Nonhistone nuclear proteins,
   phosphorylation, 33
Nucleus, 20, 23, 24, 26, 34, 37, 88,
      108, 136, 137, 139, 185,
      191-194
Nutritional changes, 56, 63

O

Ornithine decarboxylase, 68, 69
Ovary,
   carcinoma, 35
Oviduct, 89, 90, 93, 94, 121, 122

P

Pancreas, 58
Papain, 57
Parotid(s), 61, 90, 91, 192
pH, 161
Phages, 100
Phenobarbital, 117
Phorbol myristate acetate, 68
Physarum polycephalum, 27, 32, 121
Phytohemagglutinin, 7, 22, 56, 67,
      69, 89, 95, 120, 121,
      152, 154, 178
Pilocarpine, 91, 118
Plant lectins, 150
Plasmapheresis, 142
Polyamines, 68, 69
Polynucleotide ligase, 21, 22
Polyoma virus, 56, 79, 148, 150
Polyribosomes, 47, 100, 140, 141
Poly U, 141
Prereplicative phase, 53, 61, 63, 65,
   66
Progesterone, 120, 122, 196
Prolactin, 58
Pronase, 71, 155

Prophage, P2, 210
Prostate, 58, 69, 89, 120
Protease(s), 132, 135, 148, 155, 169
    inhibitors, 135
Protein(s), (see also Nonhistone
        chromosomal proteins,
        Nonhistone nuclear
        proteins)
    DNA-binding, 181
    kinases, 114, 133, 134
    synthesis, 37, 45, 47, 62, 69,
        72, 81, 118
    microtubular, 25
    nuclear, 108, 113, 134, 136,
        137, 171, 185
Puromycin, 112, 155, 197

R

2RA cells, 154, 182, 183, 212
R2 cells, 8
Rabbit lens, 180
Rabbit kidney cells, 81
Rectum,
    crypt cells, 13
Replicons, 24, 26
Ribonucleoproteins, 108, 109
Ribonucleotide reductase, 22
Ribosomes, 37, 122, 142, 181
RNA, 72·
    messenger, 37, 38, 45, 49, 54,
        71, 88, 100, 101, 140,
        142,
    nuclear, 100
    polymerase, 21, 38, 83, 86-88,
        90, 92, 100, 114, 132
    polymerase I, 100
    polymerase II, 100, 196
    ribosomal, 23, 49, 54, 63, 64,
        66, 69, 71, 79, 84, 87,
        122, 186, 197

    synthesis, 26-28, 32, 33, 38,
        39, 44, 45, 47, 50, 69,
        72, 81-84, 100, 109, 111,
        112, 139, 141
    transfer, 54
RNase, 90, 132
RNA species, 99
RNA/DNA hybridization, 70
Rous sarcoma virus, 56, 121, 149

S

S phase, 3-5, 7, 8, 13, 14, 17-19, 22-
    28, 38, 45, 46, 60, 66,
    68, 110, 177, 203, 204
Salivary gland, 7, 55, 58-60, 62, 64,
    65, 67, 68, 70, 82, 83,
    89-91, 112, 117, 120,
    124, 131, 133, 143, 177,
    178, 180, 191, 192
Sea urchin, 121, 140
Serum, 57, 67, 72, 89, 91, 92, 94-96,
    118, 120, 121, 138, 141,
    154, 156, 163-166, 182
Sialic acid, 36
Sialyl-transferase, 148
Skin, 34, 58
    carcinoma, 13, 37
Small intestine, 2, 5, 35, 177
Somatomedin, 166
Sperm cells, 113
Spermatogenesis, 87, 111
Spleen, 13, 27, 58
Stomach,
    carcinoma, 13
Sulfate,
    heparin, 151
Synchronization of cells, 17, 18
SV-40, 11, 56, 100, 120, 139, 147,
    148, 164, 182, 183, 209,
    211

T

T4 Phage, 79
3T3 cells, 22, 56, 61, 67, 79, 83, 95,
        147, 150-154, 156, 163-
        165, 171
3T6 cells, 49, 92, 154, 165, 182, 183
Testosterone, 89
Tetraploid cells, 8, 40
Thymidine kinase, 22, 47, 60, 61
Thymidylate synthetase, 22, 60, 61
Thymus, 85, 94, 95, 110, 123
Tobacco mosaic virus, 122
Trachea, 13, 27
Transferrin, 63
Triiodothyronine, 58, 114, 168
Trout testes, 87, 111
Trypsin, 57, 66, 152, 154-156, 165
Tumor(s), 12, 13, 50
        growth, 10, 11
        cells, 33, 36, 44
Tyrosine aminotransferase, 47, 139,
        140

U

Ultraviolet light, 207, 208
Uterus, (see also Estrogens) 7, 55, 58,
        63, 85, 89, 120, 154,
        183, 196

Uterine epithelium, 50

V

Vicia faba, 2

W

Wheat germ agglutinin, 36, 148, 150,
        151
Wool follicles, 50

X

Xenopus laevis, 6, 87, 136, 137
Xeroderma pigmentosum, 206-208,
        210

Y

Yeast, 14, 39, 40, 70, 79

Z

Zn^{++}, 56, 57